Dynamic memory

Dynamic memory

A theory of reminding and learning in computers and people

ROGER C. SCHANK
Yale University

CAMBRIDGE UNIVERSITY PRESS

Cambridge
London   New York   New Rochelle
Melbourne   Sydney

To Diane

Published by the Press Syndicate of the University of Cambridge
The Pitt Building, Trumpington Street, Cambridge CB2 1RP
32 East 57th Street, New York, NY 10022, USA
296 Beaconsfield Parade, Middle Park, Melbourne 3206, Australia

© Cambridge University Press 1982

First published 1982

Printed in the United State of America

Library of Congress Cataloging in Publication Data

Schank, Roger C., 1946–
Dynamic memory.

Includes index.
1. Memory. 2. Learning, Psychology of.
3. Artificial intelligence. 4. Comprehension.
I. Title

BF371.S36 001.53′5 82-1353 AACR2

ISBN 0 521 24858 2 hard covers
ISBN 0 521 27029 4 paperback

Contents

Foreword

ROBERT P. ABELSON

When Roger Schank and I wrote *Scripts, Plans, Goals, and Understanding* (SPGU) in 1977, it was a benchmark for us. The trails beyond that benchmark were uncharted, but we had a very good sense of where we had come from, and which new directions seemed worth pursuing. The present book represents one of those new directions, one that Roger has picked out to explore.

I am not a co-author on this one. Roger has run ahead along the trail on his own initiative. Nevertheless, we have had numerous conversations about the topics of this book, and he has asked me to write this foreword to give my perspective.

SPGU was an odd book. It was mainly about artificial intelligence programs for understanding texts about mundane human activities, but it also made some psychological claims – claims which had not been tested by psychological research in the standard fashion to which experimental psychologists were accustomed. There were, we explained, reasons for this. The necessity for experimental controls often imposes a task framework which seems unnatural to the process being studied, and may encourage unwanted strategic behavior on the part of the subjects. For example, in studying the processes which a reader uses on-line in story comprehension, the psychologist inclines either toward using short, fragmentary passages, or if the stimuli are longer, then toward interrupting the subject frequently during reading to pose some reaction time task. Pretty soon the subject may start anticipating and preparing for what he needs to do at the next interruption, hardly the mental mode that normally obtains.

The fussbudget demands of well-controlled experimental procedure are not *necessarily* fatal to the integrity of natural processes. There is now a great variety of methods for the study of cognitive functions, and some of them may minimize obtrusiveness. But it takes many years of research to develop efficient, powerful, bug-free experimental tools.

At the time we wrote SPGU, we weren't willing to wait for psychological techniques to catch up to the level at which we were conceptualizing. At various phases of the writing process, I would worry about the lack of data pertinent to this or that idea, but Roger persistently argued that if we waited for experimental developments, we would never get our system down on paper. This was clearly an appropriate argument, and the publication of data-thin SPGU did not in fact set psychology back a hundred years. Instead, SPGU generated a great deal of interest and helped (along with other developments in cognitive science) promote a rash of pertinent experiments.

How did we manage to get away with this violation of established psychological canons? I think that three factors were involved. First, the strictly psychological claims we made were quite modest, and they were supportable by several converging lines of argument. Our essential message was that human text comprehension necessarily involves the use of high-level knowledge structures which serve to generate expectations about what is coming next. This is not such a revolutionary message, or even now a highly debatable one, but in 1977 it was very useful to say it and to amplify it with the possible details of a number of particular types of knowledge structures.

Second, we used a methodology alternative to psychological experimentation, a methodology which was adequate to our purpose at the time. Our main purpose was to show that certain structural possibilities had to exist in any decently functioning comprehension system, and we used contrasting linguistic stimulus examples. That is, we would present pairs of sentences that created a coherent impression, and altered pairs producing incoherence, and we would ask what it was that the reader would have to know in order to be privy to the impression of coherence when it occurred. Such a method is very familiar to linguists but unfamiliar to psychologists. It is very weak if one wishes to know how a given cognitive process works, but it is very persuasive in demonstrating structural necessities, for example, that scripts or things very much like scripts have to be available to the human understander. And that was the kind of thing we wanted to show.

Third, we were quite explicitly tentative about claims at the detailed level. We did not insist that the themes or goal types or planboxes we outlined were the only possibilities, merely that they were useful for artificial intelligence applications and that alternative outlines would probably take similar form. As for processing details, we made few serious claims. It was clear, for example, that the way that the SAM program used scripts was not a realistic or sensible psychological model.

The net result of provoking interest in high-level knowledge structures has been to focus a lot of experimental effort on precisely those issues of detail which were not really addressed in SPGU. Experimental cognitive psychologists have been struggling to articulate the properties of script and plan structures (Abbott, Black, & Smith, 1982; Bower, Black, & Turner, 1979; Galambos, 1981; Galambos & Black, 1981; Graesser, Gordon, & Sawyer, 1979; Graesser, Woll, Kowalski, & Smith, 1980) and to understand the processes involved in the comprehension, summarization, and recall of story materials (Abbott & Black, 1982; Black & Bern, 1981; Black & Bower, 1980; Freedle, 1979; Graesser, 1981; Just & Carpenter, 1977; Kintsch & van Dijk, 1978; Lehnert, Black, & Reiser, 1981; Reiser & Black, 1982; Reiser, Lehnert, & Black, 1981). Some of this work is being carried out in the Yale Cognitive Science Program (Abbott & Black, 1982; Abbott, Black, & Smith, 1982; Black & Bern, 1981; Galambos & Black, 1981; Reiser, Lehnert, & Black, 1981) and will be systematically reported in a separate volume.

Now Roger Schank has plunged off in a new direction, reported in the present book. Some people may wistfully have hoped that experimental psychologists were catching up to artificial intelligencers so as to work in parallel on a shared agenda, and they will be shaken by this book. Roger deals to some extent with previous issues, such as the relationship between similar scripts and what that implies about how script-based knowledge is really organized (in the process departing from what was said in SPGU). But in the main he is breaking new territory and making a host of new claims. Testing these will require yet more new methodological development and a determined research effort.

This book is *not* about artificial intelligence. It is explicitly psychological. It is about how memory for experiences is organized, and how memory can *automatically* change and grow so that intelligent profit is made from past experiences. True, programs can be written to take advantage of the book's ideas, and programs at Yale are indeed starting to appear containing MOPs and TOPs, two of the exotic structural creatures featured in the book. But the excitement of the enterprise comes mainly from its promise as a psychological theory.

A central role is played by the everyday phenomenon of *reminding*. Why does one experience remind us of another, Schank asks, especially in the intriguing case when the two experiences share little apparent similarity of surface content. It must be because the second experience – the *reminding* – is a natural product of the attempt to understand the first, he asserts. Thus each reminding experience can serve as a kind of fingerprint to the identity of the corresponding understanding mechanism.

When Roger first had this insight, he badgered all his colleagues and students to report interesting reminding experiences to him. Psychologists unfortunately have not studied spontaneous remindings, instead confining their study of memory to the more directed and directable phenomena of recall and recognition. (This is the way it goes in psychology: if something is hard to control experimentally, it tends not to get studied.) So Roger had to gather his own data – of a case example, not an experimental, sort. Many people at Yale became specialists at catching fleeting examples from their own thinking, and from the reports of these reminding mavens come most of the examples in this book. I believe that they do not differ systematically from examples that occur in individuals innocent of their theoretical significance, but on this point, the reader of the present and the data of the future can be the judges.

Readers will differ in how much they like this book. It is written in a breathless style, rife with circumlocutions and ellipses. It is assertive beyond the norms of the cautious, scholarly scientist. Some of these assertions are wrong, although in deference to the norms of foreword writing, I'm not going to tell you which ones they are. That would prejudice your own evaluation of Schank's claims as you go along – and besides, I'm not sure myself (although I have some guesses). On the plus side you will find a powerfully intuitive mind turned loose on a set of fascinating questions, questions that will occupy a central place in the cognitive science of the next decade. The ideas are sweeping and important, and for every one that is wrong, there are two or three that are right.

If you lie back and relax as you read, you will expose yourself to a great deal of insight. On the other hand, you may not be willing or able to do this. As I try to imagine a possible negative reaction to this book, I am reminded (*sic*) of a personal experience:

As a teenager, I was a camp counselor for a group of seven- and eight-year-old children. They differed among themselves, of course, on all the dimensions along which human beings can vary, but one especially noteworthy child was an intensely serious youngster named Steven. He was very bright, and very knowledgeable about things scientific, but he had trouble getting into things and enjoying himself. The counselors were continually trying to devise ways to improve the quality of Steven's social and emotional experience.

One week my Aunt Sara, the Head Counselor, organized a breakfast hike for the children. Everybody got up before dawn and hiked with flashlights up to a secret and special location known as The Ledge, a magnificent spot from which the entire horizon beyond the neighboring hills could be seen. Soon the dawn began to break, and a great red orb appeared on the skyline. "Look, children, look," said Aunt Sara with warmth and enthusiasm, "the sun is rising!"

Everyone fell silent, transfixed, staring eastward. Then the silence was broken by a dry, young voice. "The Sun never rises," said Steven. "It's the Earth that goes around the Sun."

Preface

One of the most frustrating and at the same time tantalizing things about working in Artificial Intelligence is that you are never done. It is even difficult after working for a long time on a book and finally completing it, to have a sense of accomplishment. It is always clear that there are many problems with what one has written. It is often less clear just where those problems are. But, it is always certain that as the ideas proposed are worked into computer programs, only their bare bones will remain the same. The substance of one's idea is quite likely to continue to change as the experimentation points up the initial problems.

When Bob Abelson and I finished *Scripts, Plans, Goals, and Understanding,* we knew that the work was seriously incomplete. Our choice was to wait for it to be complete, which might have taken a very long time, or to publish it then and take the consequences. The consequences of publishing it when we did were quite pleasant actually. Many workers in psychology and other disciplines took our book in the vein that it was intended, as a set of suggestions for how experimentation might proceed.

This current work is intended in a similar vein. It had its origins in the incompleteness of Schank and Abelson. We knew, when we wrote that book, that we had not provided adequate definitions for some of the notions we were developing. In particular, we knew that the concept of a script, while intuitively attractive, needed a great deal more consideration than we had given it. The point of that work was that such knowledge structures were a natural part of language understanding. That having been shown, we left the myriad residual issues that followed from that hypothesis to others.

One of those residual issues was memory. We really did not consider the consequences of our claims with respect to memory. Fortunately, others did. I had a number of conversations with Gordon Bower and Ed Smith, two psychologists who worried about the claims we were making. At the same time, I began to get increasingly concerned about the nature of the theory underlying the programs in our own laboratory. It seemed that no one really had a good idea about what the theoretical limits to a script were. If it was convenient to do so, a structure was labeled a script.

While these concerns about scripts troubled me, their consequences were not grave. What was more important to me was that a number of the programs that we were developing at Yale seemed to have the problem of being too cumbersome to be of great use. We had always argued that there are no easy shortcuts in natural language processing. Understanding requires a great deal of knowledge, but humans do not crumble from the weight of their own information store. Automated data bases on the other hand, do get overwhelmed when they *know* too much. We wanted to make sure that any understanding system we developed would be capable of acquiring, storing, and using its knowledge with some ease.

The problems we were developing were encumbered by their knowledge, however. They had no easy means of acquiring it, and storage and retrieval created massive problems. Moreover, the programs had no real sense of what they knew. They were like a librarian who can read but has no memory for what he read after a very short interval. In other words, they never got smarter.

A program should not be cast in stone, immutable and impossible to affect. It should, if it is to be a good model of a person, be changed by what it reads. It should be unpredictable in the sense that it might just know more than you thought it knew. So, in our laboratory, static programs such as FRUMP, SAM, PAM, and POLITICS began to give way to more dynamic programs, such as CYRUS and IPP. Our emphasis was on letting the purpose of the program guide what we wanted to get out of that program. IPP and CYRUS could surprise us in ways that the others could not. Of course, as any computer scientist knows, such surprises are not always pleasant.

My motivations in my work have always been a mesh of an interest in human understanding and computer understanding. When I first began to work on representing the meaning derived from natural language expressions, it became clear to me that one could never really know the *correct* representation for a sentence without knowing something of the intentions, beliefs, and general memory conditions of the understander and the speaker. (In fact, in 1971 I wrote a paper entitled, *Intention, Memory and Computer Understanding* that focused on these issues.) But it was not until the above issues started to make their presence felt that I began to seriously work on memory.

So, I became interested in memory. Bob Abelson and I discussed various issues that concerned us, and, as is my habit, I began to write.

Unfortunately for the clarity and precision of this book, Abelson became involved in other matters and never did get to writing his part of this book as we had originally planned. What is here is not entirely mine however. In the early stages of writing this book, I discussed many of the issues here with Bob Abelson, Janet Kolodner, Mike Lebowitz, Larry Birnbaum, Chris Riesbeck, Margot Flowers, and Gregg Collins. In addition, I presented my ideas on numerous occasions to members of the Yale AI project and received helpful ideas and comments.

The written version of this book was gone over by many of my students, former students and colleagues. Mike Lebowitz, Jerry Feldman, Drew McDermott, Chris Riesbeck, Bob Abelson, Andrew Ortony, and Jaime Carbonell provided helpful comments on various drafts of this book. A few of my students worked long and hard at attempting to get this work into more clearly understandable English than I normally write. I'd like to especially thank Larry Birnbaum, Gregg Collins, Larry Hunter, Kris Hammond, and Margot Flowers for helping me with the final draft of the book.

No book can be written without the help and consideration of the people who interact with you daily. During most of the course of writing this book I was Chairman of the Computer Science Department at Yale. Stephen Slade took over a great many of the duties of that job allowing me to write. Linda Fusco protected me from the outside world, letting me think without interruption when all around her was incredibly hectic. Ann Drinan ran the International Joint Conference on Artificial Intelligence of which I was Program Chairman during the period that I was working on this book. Patti Oronzo worked on preparing the manuscript, with the advice of Margot Flowers. And, finally, Diane Schank kept my life carefree and warm. I cannot imagine how I would have been able to complete this book without the help of these good people. I sincerely thank them all.

Woodbridge, Connecticut   Roger C. Schank
October, 1981

1 Introduction to dynamic memory

What is a dynamic memory? It is a flexible, open-ended system. Compare the way an expert stores knowledge about books in his field to the way a library catalog system does the same job. In a library, an initial set of categories is decided upon to describe a domain of knowledge. Various boxes are then used to record the titles, authors, and subjects of the books, within those categories. Such a system is not *dynamic*. Eventually, the categories will have to be changed. They will require updating, as certain categories become overutilized. Other categories will have to be created to handle subjects and subject divisions unthought of at the time of the initial definition of the categories.

A library does not have a dynamic memory. It changes with great difficulty. Most importantly, to change it requires outside intervention. An expert has neither of these problems. He can change his internal classification system easily when his interests change, or when his knowledge of the subject matter changes. An expert is a self-conscious being. He knows when he knows something, and he can make observations about what he knows. He can thus alter the memory structures that catalog what he knows if the need arises. He has a dynamic memory.

In a library, categories are not the only problem. Libraries require physical space. Building and floor space must be allocated to various subject areas. The initial conception of the physical layout of the library might have ignored an area of knowledge that the library later came to specialize in; or, an entire floor might have been devoted to a subject in anticipation of a collection that never materialized. Knowing where you want to put a book, or information about this book, requires having some preconception of the possible places available. Such decisions can only be made on the basis of prior experience. New experiences will show early classifications to be wrong in initial conception. In other words, we cannot always know in what way information we receive may turn out to be valuable at some later time.

1

The problem for libraries in this regard is no doubt great. People, on the other hand, seem to be able to cope with new information with ease. We can find a place for new information in our memories. We can find old information, too. We can learn from a multiplicity of common experiences. Our memories change dynamically in the way they store information by abstracting significant generalizations from our experiences and storing the exceptions to those generalizations. They do all this without an outside observer, who, in the case of the library, can decide that a given cataloging scheme is out of date. Humans are not aware of their own cataloging schemes. They are just capable of using them.

Consciousness does not extend to an awareness of how we encode or retrieve experiences. Our dynamic memories seem to organize themselves in such a way as to be able to adjust their initial encodings of the world to reflect growth and new understanding. Our memories are structured in a way that allows us to learn from our experiences. They can reorganize to reflect new generalizations – in a way a kind of automatic catagorization scheme – that can be used to process new experiences on the basis of old ones. In short, our memories dynamically adjust to reflect our experiences. A dynamic memory is one that can change its own organization when new experiences demand it. A dynamic memory can learn.

Background

The research in Artificial Intelligence at our laboratory at Yale University has been focused primarily on the problem of getting computers to be able to read. We have made a certain amount of progress. (See Cullingford, 1977; DeJong, 1977; Dyer & Lehnert, 1980; Wilensky, 1978 for descriptions of some of our programs that read text.)

But no computer program that fails to remember what it has just read can honestly be said to be comprehending. We have tried, during the course of our work in creating computer programs that understand language, to avoid the memory problem. But, the separation of language and memory is undoubtedly artificial and probably impossible. People know, after reading a story a few times, that they have read the story before. People get bored and irritated by being asked to read something again and again, but our computer programs never did. The programs did not have memories that were attempting to gather information from what they read. They were merely trying to cope with the problems of language.

Language is a memory-based process, however. Language is a medium by which thoughts in a memory are transmitted to another memory, one of several vehicles used for the transmission of information to memory.

All of the senses can affect memory. Language is an encoding of one kind of sense data. It seems obvious that any theory of language must refer to, and be a subpart of, a theory of memory.

In our previous work, we attempted to provide some view of how memory might represent information about events. In Schank and Abelson (1977), we developed the notion of a script, evolved from earlier versions (Abelson 1973 & 1976). We said there that a script was a kind of data structure that was useful in the processing of text to the extent that it directed the inference process and tied together pieces of input. Input sentences were connected together by referring to the overall structure of the script to which they made reference. Thus, scripts were, in our view, a kind of high level knowledge structure that could be called upon to supply background information during the understanding process. Scripts, as embodied in the computer programs that we wrote, were essentially sets of predictions of event sequences. A script was constituted as a list of events that comprise a stereotypical episode. Input events that matched one or more of the events in the list would cause the program to infer that the other events in the list had also taken place.

Since our book was written, some psychological experiments have found the notion of a script useful in explaining the behavior of children (McCartney & Nelson, 1981; Nelson, 1979; Nelson & Gruendel, 1979), and adults (Bower, 1978; Graesser, Gordon, & Sawyer, 1979; Graesser, Woll, Kowalski, & Smith, 1980; Jebousek, 1978; Smith, Adams, & Schorr, 1978), engaged in the language comprehension process. Thus, some of the representations we proposed have psychological validity (Abelson, 1980; Graesser, 1981).

When language is viewed as a memory process, one's overall view of how understanding works must change somewhat. Thus, our view of various parts of the language comprehension process has evolved somewhat in the last few years. We have begun to recognize, for example, that language understanding is an integrated process. Our early models were modular in nature. For example, SAM (our original story comprehension program) had a modular organization (Cullingford, 1978). After translating a sentence into Conceptual Dependency (the meaning representation scheme devised by Schank, 1972), SAM began the process of script application. (Script application involves the recognition that a given script applies in a situation. When a script has been successfully identified, the result is that a set of predictions are made about what events are likely to transpire.) We knew that such a modular approach was unrealistic (surely we begin to understand what a sentence is about before the sentence is completely uttered). We built SAM in a modular fashion because that was the easiest way to work out the mechanics of script application. To do this, it was easiest to divorce the parsing process from script application. But scripts are the sources of memories. How we understand is affected by what is in our memories. That is, language understanding is different when there are different memory structures controlling the process. A coherent theory of the structures in memory must naturally precede a complete theory of language understanding.

To solve various problems involved in building understanding systems, we need to look at the problem of the kinds of high level knowledge structures available in the understanding process. What else is there available to an understanding system besides scripts? In PAM (Wilensky, 1978) and POLITICS (Carbonell, 1979) we used plans and goals as high level structures that control understanding. Certainly any memory must have access to such structures. But how many different sources of predictions are there? How can we find out what the various memory structures are like?

Recall that we are interested in more than just good understanding systems. We want systems that *learn* as well. Further, and perhaps most important, we want to understand how the human mind processes experiences. We want to know how it copes with new information and derives new knowledge from that information. To do all this we need a coherent theory of adaptable memory structures – in other words, a dynamic memory.

A dynamic memory would have to have some way of structuring its knowledge. At the same time, it would have to have some way of altering the structures that it previously found useful, when their value faded. It is unlikely that high level structures in memory are innate. The high level structures that develop in the memories of people develop because they address the needs that arise during processing by the understander. That is, what an understander needs to do to process the experiences he has will affect the development of structures in his memory.

Scripts revisited

In this book we will develop a theory of the high level memory structures that comprise a dynamic memory. That theory has its base in the theory of processing natural language that was developed in Schank and Abelson (1977). One key problem that we will deal with in this book is how the process of abstraction and generalization from experience works. Previously, we had suggested that *scripts,* and other structures, were part of this process. We endeavored to find out what kinds of structures might be available for use in processing. In general, we ignored the problems of the development of such structures, the ability of the proposed structures to change themselves, and the problems of retrieval and storage of information posed by those structures. We concentrated instead on processing issues. But, because of the lack of cohesion of all of the relevant issues in the design of our theory, many of the high level structures that we suggested were poorly defined. In particular, the notion of a script, an idea that has been widely explored in the literature, has been used by many researchers to mean nearly anything.

The term has been used to describe a variety of different phenomena. What one psychologist has meant by the term is not necessarily what another has meant by it. To further confuse the issue, even within our group at Yale, there has been widely different usage of the term.

The issue of the correct application of a particular piece of terminology is of course of little significance. But, in this case there are some important theoretical issues at stake. Scripts have been taken to mean *some high level knowledge source* and thus, given that there are probably a great many varieties of possible knowledge sources, different claims have been made for scripts that on occasion conflict with one another. In our own research we have differentiated between plans and scripts, for example, but that distinction has not always been clear. Frequently when we presented the issue of plans and goals we were asked why *robbing a liquor store* was a plan and not a script or why *reading the Michelin Guide* was not a script. The line between scripts and plans seemed fuzzy. For *liquor store robbing* to be a script and not a plan it would have had to have been done a great many times. Of course such a thing might very well be a script for some people. We had chosen it as an instance of a plan because we were trying to illustrate the process of plan application, which was very different in nature from that of script application. In plan application, inferences about goals are made in order to establish the connections between input actions and the achievement of some goal. The most important point about script application is that often such goal-related inferences cannot be made. For example, without knowledge of the Japanese restaurant script there is no way to determine why a customer took off his shoes.

The difference, then, between scripts and plans resides in the kinds of interconnections that one is trying to make. The less one knows about a situation, the less familiar one is with a certain kind of situation, the more inference work one has to do in order to process inputs dealing with that situation. Using scripts involves less work; planning implies more work. The real difference between SAM and PAM was how much work, and the kind of work, that needed to be done in using these different knowledge sources.

Nevertheless, the feeling persisted that a strong theoretical distinction between scripts and plans, or for that matter between scripts and any other high level knowledge structure, was not all that clear. Our initial definition of a script was "a structure that describes an appropriate sequence of events in a particular context" or "a predetermined stereotyped sequence of actions that defines a well-known situation" (Schank & Abelson, 1975). In Schank and Abelson, we stated that there were three kinds of scripts: situational, personal, and instrumental. The archetype that used scripts was SAM (Cullingford, 1978; Schank, 1975), a program intended to understand stories that used restaurants as their background.

Restaurant stories being neither plentiful nor very interesting, we began to look for new domains after we had initially demonstrated the power of script-based processing. We chose car accidents because of their ubiquity and essential simplicity and began to alter SAM to handle these. Immediately we ran into the problem of what exactly a script was. Is there a *car accident* script? Clearly, people who have never been in a car accident would not have a car accident script in the same sense that they might be said to have a restaurant script. Certainly the method of acquisition would be vastly different. Furthermore, the ordered step-by-step nature of a script, that is, its essential stereotypical nature due to common cultural convention, was different.

This was emphasized in the way that a car accident script actually could be used to handle newspaper stories. Whenever a car accident occurred, we had to expect that an ambulance script, a hospital emergency room script, a police report, and possibly a subsequent trial script, and maybe others as well, might also be present. Were all these things scripts? And, if they were, why was it that they seemed so different from the restaurant script in acquisition, use, and predictive power? To put it another way, it seemed all right to say that people know that in a restaurant you can either read a menu and order or go stand in line for your food. We felt justified in saying that there were many different *tracks* to a restaurant script, but that each of these tracks was essentially a form of the larger script. That is, they were like each other in important ways and might be expected to be stored with each other within the same overall outer structure in memory.

But what of accidents? Was there a general accident script of which collisions, accidental shootings, and falling out of windows were different tracks? Alternatively, was there a vehicle accident script of which those involving cars, trucks, and motorcycles were different tracks? Or was there a car accident script of which one car hitting an obstruction, two cars colliding, and chain reactions were different tracks?

It turned out for the purpose of creating SAM that none of this mattered. We encoded it all as scripts and allowed certain scripts to fire off other scripts to handle the sequence, accident, ambulance, emergency room, and so on. The fact that we could make it work on a computer this way is basically irrelevant to the issue of the ultimate form and place of scripts, however. Did the fact that it worked in SAM really suggest that for people the emergency room script is in some important way a part of the car accident script? Although the idea of a general accident script seems to contradict an experientially based definition of scripts, that would have worked in SAM as well.

Gradually then, a practical definition of scripts was beginning to emerge that bore only surface similarity to the theoretical notion of scripts as a knowledge source for controlling inferences and tying together texts in highly constrained and stereotypical domains. This practical definition was that a script was a data structure that was a useful source of predictions. Scripts were supposed to depend on issues related to development based on repeated experience. But our use of scripts was not in agreement with our theory.

Whenever a script was accessed and an initial pattern match for an input made, the script could be used to predict what was coming next, or to take what did come next and place it within the overall pattern. By script, then, in SAM'S terms, we meant a gigantic pattern that could be matched partially in a piecemeal fashion.

This problem of defining scripts precisely became even more difficult when work began on FRUMP (DeJong, 1977). FRUMP is a program that was intended as a practical script-based approach to story understanding. SAM was rather slow and exceedingly fragile, since it made every inference within a script that was there to be made and in doing so had to rely upon an immense vocabulary and world knowledge store. Because the stories that were to be read by SAM came from the newspapers, an unexpected vocabulary item was not only possible, it was rather likely. SAM had very little ability to recover from problems caused by missing vocabulary or missing world knowledge. (A program was designed to take care of this to some extent, however, Granger 1977.)

FRUMP got around these problems by relying more heavily on the predictive nature of scripts and less heavily on what the text actually said. FRUMP does not actually parse the input it receives. Rather, it predicts what it will see and goes about looking for words, phrases, or meanings that substantiate its predictions. To do this, FRUMP relies upon what we termed *sketchy scripts*. Examples of sketchy scripts include earthquakes, breaking diplomatic relations, wars, arson, and snowstorms. In other words, nearly anything at all could be considered a sketchy script (including, of course, robbing a liquor store, which put us back to square one). The theoretical difference between SAM'S scripts and FRUMP'S sketchy scripts is negligible. FRUMP'S scripts, from this point of view, are simply shorter and contain less information.

Actually, FRUMP'S scripts are essentially just a set of requests (Riesbeck, 1975), which is another way of saying that they constitute a set of predictions about what might happen, and a set of rules about what to assume if those predictions are or are not fulfilled. But the concept of a script as an organized set of predictions is not exactly what we had in mind by the notion originally. It is easy to see why for FRUMP earthquakes and breaking diplomatic relations can be scripts.

But if earthquakes are scripts, then what is a script, anyway? Few of us have ever actually been in an earthquake; even fewer of us have actually broken diplomatic relations. But we do have knowledge about such events that can be used to understand stories about such things or to handle situations similar in nature to those events. This knowledge can be encoded as a set of rules about what happens in general in disasters, or in negative relationships between countries. Are such sets of rules scripts? They are the rules FRUMP uses when it uses sketchy scripts. So perhaps the problem is just terminological. Perhaps the whole issue can be resolved by renaming sketchy scripts to be, say, *knowledge packets*. By this reasoning, many of SAM'S scripts would be knowledge packets as well. What would be left?

A great deal of what would be left would be knowledge that looks a lot like planning information. What is a *knowledge packet* about negative relations between countries? To a large extent it is precisely the knowledge of methods that one can use when one wants to deal with someone else in a negative way, where that knowledge has been abstracted in such a way as to be relevant to international relations. Similarly, outside of the knowledge specifically associated with car accidents (e.g., that crashes can be caused by drunk drivers; that the police will file an accident report), most of the relevant knowledge in a car accident is true in any serious accident or, in fact, in any negative physical event.

The distinction then, between scripts and other high level knowledge structures hinges upon the notions of abstraction and generalization. Scripts were considered by us to be specific information associated with specific situations. The original emphasis on a script being a source of information, naturally acquired by having undergone an experience many times, depended on the notion of a script as a very specific set of sequential facts about a very specific situation.

On the other side of the coin, people have general information associated with general situations such as negative relationships between countries or natural physical disasters. This general information is very likely related to specific script-related information. The usual method of acquisition of script-based information is direct repeated experience, but people acquire general information in a more complex fashion – by abstracting and generalizing from multiple experiences and from the experiences of others.

In addition, if there are two diffent kinds of information in memory, specific structures based directly upon experience, and general structures containing more abstract information, it follows that the methods of storage in memory and retrieval from memory for both kinds of structures might be different as well. In comprehending the breaking of diplomatic relations, we can use information stored under the historical relationship between two countries, their position in the world political situation, their economic relationship, as well as information about what individuals do when they are angered or want to protest another's actions and so on. Such information cannot logically be stored in any one place in memory. Rather, it must be derived from multiple sources by many different retrieval methods. To not do this, to have all this information stored in only one location, is to have a script.

The difference, then, between a script-based memory and a memory based upon more general structures, is that in the first case what we know in a given situation comes from what we have experienced in more or less identical situations. Using more general structures allows us to make use of information originally garnered from one situation to help us in a quite different situation. General knowledge structures save space and make information experienced in one situation available for use in another. One disadvantage of the script-based method is its lack of usability in similar but nonidentical situations. Reliance upon scripts inhibits learning from experience.

But, on the other hand, scripts have an advantage. We do have knowledge that is specific to particular situations. People can remember individual experiences and use those experiences to help them in processing similar experiences. Generalized information that eliminates particular differences will lose information, and such information may be valuable.

In summary then, we can say that in the computer implementation of any knowledge-based understanding system, any given set of facts can be stored in either a script-based or non-script-based form. If we choose to give up generalizability, we buy efficiency in the short term. Knowing a great deal about the domain we are in, and that domain only, will work for any system that need never transcend the boundaries of a given domain. Any *knowing system* must be able to know a great deal about one domain without losing the power to apply generalizations drawn from that knowledge to a different domain.

To correctly ascertain the proper place for scripts in a theory of natural language processing, we must first ask ourselves what human memory is like, how it got that way, and why it functions the way it does. From this perspective we can more effectively determine the relevance and place of scripts.

Generalized scripts

Before we begin our examination of issues in memory from a purely observational perspective, there is a piece of psychological evidence derived from more conventional experimental methods that bears on what we shall have to say. This work was done by Bower, Black and Turner (1979). For our purposes, in addition to showing that script-like considerations are relevant in story understanding, one of the most valuable things to come out of that work was a problem it presented for us. Recognition confusions were found by Bower et al. to occur between stories that called upon similar scripts, such as visits to the dentist and visits to the doctor. In no intuitive sense can this result be called surprising, since most people have experienced such confusions. It seems plain that in order to confuse doctor visits and dentist visits, some structure in memory is used by both stories during processing. However, if we posit a *visit to a health care professional* script in order to explain the confusion, we will have created an entity that has considerable drawbacks. In our original terms, such an entity could not be considered to be a script because scripts are supposed to reflect knowledge derived from specific experiences in specific situations. To form the **health care professional** script, the general parts of some similar scripts would have to have been abstracted out and stored at some higher level. Such a suggestion plays havoc with the original idea of a script.

The assumption here is that scripts are not merely useful data structures for processing, but that they are memory structures as well. As a memory structure, we might ask why, if we used the dentist script (hence *$DENTIST*) to interpret a relevant story, the remembrance of the story would get confused with one that used *$DOCTOR*. After all, different structures used in processing ought not to get confused with each other.

But if we assume that some structure that was a superset of those two was used, e.g., *$HEALTH CARE VISIT,* such a structure would not account for the possible confusion of a dentist story with a visit to an accountant's office. It might be that an even more abstract structure such as *$OFFICE VISIT* was being used, but that kind of entity is getting more and more separated from any specific experience or reasonably grouped set of experiences. If information is stored at such a high level of abstraction, then understanding a story becomes much more complex than we had initially imagined. We cannot get away with simply applying the most relevant script, even in what appear to be very stereotyped and script-based situations, because a great many entities such as *$OFFICE VISIT* are likely to be relevant at one time.

If we can get confused between events that occurred in a dentist visit and those that occurred in a visit to an accountant's office, then the phenomenon observed by Bower et al. is too complex to handle by invented generalized scripts such as *$HEALTH CARE VISIT.* On the other hand, we are certainly not storing new inputs about dentists in terms of a visit to an accountant. One possibility is that there is no dentist script in memory in the form we had previously suggested. At the same time, generalized scripts such as *$HEALTH CARE VISIT* probably do not exist either.

Before we attempt to broach the question of what is the correct kind of memory structure, it is important to realize that any solution we propose must be formulated in human memory terms. Clearly one can construct a program that uses a dentist script to understand stories where a dentist's office is the background context. That is not the issue. The issue is one of extensibility. Just because one can construct a program to do something in a particular way using a particular method does not indicate that that program will be naturally extensible. If the program is not naturally extensible, then it is unlikely to have much value as a psychological theory. Its only value as a program is as a test for the viability of its basic notions as process models (or as a program with practical value if that turns out to be the case). So henceforth we will evaluate the notion of scripts in memory terms, rather than considering their value in a program. Furthermore, we shall consider scripts and other memory structures, from the point of view of their ability to change through experience. A script, and any other memory structure, must be part of a dynamic memory. Any structure proposed for memory must be capable of self-modification. If it is not, then we must question its psychological validity. Thus, when we ask if there is a dentist script, we mean to ask: Is there one unique structure in human memory directly containing the information necessary for processing a story about a visit to a dentist? And, if such a structure does exist, what is the method by which such a structure would be modified as a result of experiences relevant to that structure but not completely predicted by it?

Levels of memory

To attempt to answer this question, we must examine the kinds of information that need to be stored in memory together with the likely methods of storing that information. The overall issue here is the level of generality in terms of what information is stored. We must ascertain what the most economical storage scheme is and whether such a scheme is likely to have psychological plausibility.

To start, therefore, we ask: What kinds of things is a person likely to remember? Obviously, a person can remember in some detail, for a short period of time, a particular experience. But after a while, the details will be forgotten, unless those details were interesting or unusual in some way.

Consider a recent experience of mine. I took a trip to Palo Alto, a place I have not only traveled to many times, but also lived in for five years. During that trip, I could answer questions about what hotel I was staying in: what my room number was; how much the hotel cost; what kind of car I had rented; what color it was; what the rental car agency was; how long it took for the bus to take me to the rental car agency; and so on. In short, the details of the trip, even the petty details, were available immediately during or after that experience.

After a week or two, most of the details of such a trip are likely to be completely forgotten. Indeed after an hour or two, details such as what song was playing on the car radio, or the color of the rent-a-car pick-up van, were certainly forgotten. Why? How is it that some parts of the experience are forgotten and some are not?

Psychologists have differentiated between short-term memory and long-term memory. Short-term memory, however, lasts seconds, not hours. It is likely that there is a kind of intermediate-term memory that utilizes temporary memory structures. Whether an intermediate-term memory item gets retained in long-term memory depends on the significance of that item with respect to other items already retained in long-term memory. That is, we only remember what is relevant to remember. The memory of some events in an episode last forever; others are forgotten almost instantly. Clearly there is a kind of selection process at work that picks some memories for special treatment by retaining them for long-term memory. It is the nature of this selection mechanism and the nature of the types of memories that do not fade quickly that is the key problem before us.

Consider the above trip viewed from a distance of a year or more. A few particularly interesting details remain but the majority are gone. If I took many trips to Palo Alto that year then it is even more likely that the details of the above trip would be unretrievable.

Some of the details can be reconstructed, however. For example, although it may not be readily available what rental car company or what hotel was used, it is often the case that people asked to answer such questions can do so with the following kinds of reasoning:

a) I always stay at the Holiday Inn, so that's where I would have stayed.
b) There are only two rent-a-car agencies that I ever used and I had received my Hertz discount card around that time, so it would have been Hertz.
c) I can't recall the room number but I remember where it was and I could take you there (or nearly there).

Such answers are instances of what is commonly called reconstructive memory. The questions for a reconstructive view of memory are these:

1. What is actually stored in memory and how is that information stored such that reconstruction can take place?
2. What different kinds of reconstruction are there?

Clearly the three answers above require very different kinds of reconstructive capabilities. In each case the methods that effect the recall are very different and the places searched are very different.

One of the kinds of structures searched in reconstruction would seem to be those that encode a general, abstract view of how things happen in some category of events. In this way, particular instances in that category can be assumed to have followed the general rule. In our memories there are facts about certain things in general – what a hotel is like, how to rent a car, what a dentist visit is like. These facts are crucial to the reconstructing process. Or, to put it another way, these facts form an important part of our ability to remember (really reconstruct). Thus, we can recall something by recalling the prototype for that event rather than the event itself and *coloring* the general memory with whatever specifics might be available. If we ask someone to imagine driving a car or using a knife and fork, they seem to have two avenues open to them. Either they can attempt to recall an actual episode of doing this, or they can draw upon general information associated with a prototype of that event that is stored in memory. Such prototypes exist because people have experienced these events so often that they have generalized them. That is, they have forgotten specific knives, forks, plates, and so on. Even when a specific episode is chosen, the smallest details, such as the pattern on the fork, will usually not be available. Thus, with either recall approach, general memory structures are used for reconstruction.

The role of such general memory structures in processing is to understand input events by noticing that they completely match the default representation present in the general structure. When an identical match is noticed an episode can be forgotten. *Hearing the radio in the car* is so normative for some people, that is, it matches their general structure for **car driving** so well, and is of so little consequence, that it can be forgotten.

The use of such general structures in memory is twofold. First, they help us decide what to pay attention to. If an item is matched by a general structure, it is understood as being of no use to remember. On the other hand, when an experienced event differs from the general structure, its difference may be noted. Noticing and recalling differences of the same kind enables learning. We modify our old structures on the basis of mismatches. This is what a dynamic memory is all about. The process of learning by explaining expectation failures that have come from predictions encoded in high level memory structures is the subject of this book.

Finding relevant structures

We are suggesting, then, that by utilizing general structures to encode what we know in memory, we can learn, particularly if our experiences differ from those general structures. Thus, what is actually stored in long-term memory are those episodes that differ from the norm. We are further saying that, given enough differences from the norm, it is necessary to adjust our memory structures accordingly so as to begin to create new general structures that account for those differences. That is, just because an episode is new once, it does not follow that it will be forever new. Eventually we will recognize what was once novel as "old hat." To do this, we must be constantly modifying our general structures, which, as we have said, is what we mean by a dynamic memory.

Thus, we must concern ourselves with the issue of how a memory structure is changed. In order to do this, we must address the issue of how a memory structure is found to be relevant in the first place. That is, how do we decide to use a given memory structure when we read a story or undergo an experience?

To consider this problem, imagine trying to answer the question,

"When was the last time you rented a car?" It seems impossible to answer this question without asking yourself why you would have rented a car, establishing that it would probably have been on a trip, and then beginning to look for recent trips. In other words, **trips** provides a context in which to search for relevant general memory structures, while **rent a car** does not. How do we explain this? Why is **trip** a source of memories and **rent a car** not?

One possibility suggested by this is that memory contains at least two kinds of entities, structures (that contain specific memories indexed in terms of their differences from the norm in that structure) and organizers of structures. One kind of structure is a *scene*. A scene provides a physical setting that serves as the basis for reconstruction. Some organizing entity must help point out the most appropriate scene. To see what I mean by this, consider the rent-a-car example. In trying to answer a question about a rent-a-car, its color, make, or place of rental, for example, the rent-a-car scene itself is of little use. This is because the scene most specific to the renting of the car, namely the actual signing of the contract and ordering of the car in the airport, is the scene that is least likely to contain the memories relevant to answering the question of when you last rented a car. On the other hand, it would be possible to answer "What color was the form you signed?" by accessing the rent-a-car scene. One major difficulty in memory retrieval is finding the scene with the memory most relevant to the information one is seeking.

An important question, then, is: What kinds of things serve as organizers of scenes? That is, what kinds of contexts are there? In order to answer this question, it should be pointed out that a scene is likely to be ordered by using different contexts. One way to access rent-a-car information is through an organizing memory structure such as **trip**. A **trip** structure would indicate what scenes normally follow each other in a trip. **Trip** would also include in it information about hotel rooms, airports and so on. Many other organizing structures can also point to such things. Thus, whereas a hotel room is a scene, it is a scene that can be expected to be part of a great many different structures. A hotel room can be part of the hotel structure, the trip structure, the visit structure, a structure involving a place (i.e., a hotel room in Hawaii), and so on. Also, these are less physical kinds of structures of which hotel rooms can be a part; for example, arguments, business deals, triumphs, frustrations. In other words, the scene **hotel room** is likely to have specific memories included in it, but those memories can be accessed by many higher level structures.

In searching for a memory, then, we are just looking for an appropriate organizing structure. This structure provides us with a set of clues as to` what scenes to look at, and, most importantly, how to set up those scenes so that we can find what we are looking for.

The place of scripts

What, then, has happened to specific structures, namely scripts? For example, what is the dentist script and where can it be found in memory? We will suggest that there is no dentist script in memory at all, at least not in the form of a list of events of the kind we previously postulated. A more reasonable organization of memory would allow for script like structures to be embedded as standardizations of various general scenes. For example, a **waiting room** scene might have one or more standardized ways that events are normally encoded. Thus, we might expect that there is a **Doctor Jones's waiting room** script or a standardized **dentist's waiting room** script attached to the waiting room scene. When available, such scripts would make specific, detailed, expectations that override more general expectations that come from higher level scenes. We will see how this works in Chapter 6.

What we are saying, then, is that the dentist script itself does not actually exist in memory in one precompiled chunk. Rather, it, or actually its subparts, can be constructed to be used as needed from the various scenes connected with the experience of visiting a dentist. Thus, we have two kinds of information with respect to visiting a dentist. We have information about what scenes, or other general structures, comprise a trip to the dentist, and we have information about what specific colorations of each scene are made because it is a dentist's waiting room (or a particular dentist's waiting room), and not a lawyer's. Specific memories, standardized as scripts or not, are thus attached to more general memories to which they relate.

The economy of such a scheme is very important. Scenes transcend the specifics of a situation so they capture generalities. Specifics are added by other structures. The construction of wht we previously called the dentist script is actually done on demand during processing time by searching for information from general organizing structures that tell which scenes will be relevant for processing.

The main issues before us, then, are: ascertaining what high level structures are likely to be used in memory; explaining how the information contained in those structures gets used in processing new inputs and recalling old ones; explaining how the experiences that have been processed change memory. We shall now attempt to answer these questions.

Part I

Reminding and processing

2   Reminding and memory

Reminding

What are the issues a theory of memory must account for? What should any memory structure, in principle, be?

The human memory system, and hence any sensibly designed computer model of that memory system must have the ability to cope with new information in a reasonable way. Any new input that is to be processed by a memory system should cause some adjustment in that system. A dynamic memory system is one that is altered in some way by every experience it processes. A memory system that fails to learn from its experiences is unlikely to be very useful.

In addition, any good memory system must be capable of finding what it has in it. This seems to go without saying, but the issue of what to find can be quite a problem. With respect to episodic memory, that is the part of the memory system concerned with memory for events that are part of personal experience, we wish to find particular episodes in memory that are closely related to the input we are processing. But how do we define relatedness? And how do we know where to look for related episodes?

One phenomenon that sheds light on both the problem of retrieval and our ability to learn is the phenomenon of reminding. Reminding is a crucial aspect of human memory that has received little attention from researchers on memory. (For example, in a highly regarded recent book that attempts to catalog research by psychologists on memory, Crowder (1976), *reminding* does not even appear in the index as a subject that is mentioned.) Yet reminding is an everyday occurrence, a common feature of memory. We are reminded of one person by another, of one building by another and so on. But, more significant than the reminding that a physical object can cause of another physical object, is the reminding that occurs across situations. One event can remind you of another.

Why does this happen? Far from being an irrelevant artifact of memory, reminding is at the root of how we understand. It is also at the root of how we learn.

At the outset, it is important to distinguish the following broad classes of reminding since they tend to have different effects in an understanding system and must be accounted for in different ways.

1. Physical objects can remind you of other physical objects.
2. Physical objects can remind you of events.
3. Events can remind you of physical objects.
4. Events can remind you of events in the same domain.
5. Events can remind you of events in different domains.

For our purposes here, we will be concerned with the last two of these (4 and 5), because we are primarily interested in event memory. To the extent that reminding can tell us about the nature and organization of the episodic memory system, the most interesting cases would be those where, in the normal course of attempting to understand an event, we are able to find a particular event in memory that in some way relates to the processing of that event. That is, the organization of a dynamic episodic memory system depends upon the use of that system in understanding. Reminding occurs as a natural part of the process of understanding new situations in terms of previously processed situations (although it is not always obvious to us as processors exactly why a given reminding has occurred). Exactly how human memory controls processing and naturally gets reminded is the question we must address.

Why one experience reminds you of another is of primary importance to any theory of human understanding and memory. If people are reminded of things during the natural course of a conversation, or while reading, or when seeing something, then this tells us something of importance about the understanding process. Given the assumption that understanding an event means finding an appropriate place for a representation of that event in memory, reminding would indicate that a specific episode in memory has been excited or *seen* during the natural course of processing the new input. To be reminded of something we must have come across it while we were processing the new input. But, to have done this we either had to be *looking* for this reminded event or else we must have *run into it accidentally*. In either case, reminding reveals something significant about the nature of memory structures and the understanding process.

If we found an episode because we were looking for it, we must ask ourselves how we knew of that episode's existence so that we were able to look for it.

If the explanation of reminding is that we *accidentally run into an episode,* we must ask why that *accident* occurs, and whether that accident has relevance to our processing.

We will argue here that it is an amalgamation of these two explanations that provides us with the method by which reminding takes place. We are not consciously looking for a particular episode in memory during processing, because we do not explicitly know of that episode's existence. We do however, know where episodes like the one we are currently processing are likely to be stored. Further, our method of processing new episodes is to utilize memory structures that contain episodes that are the most closely related to that new episode. Thus, reminding occurs when we have found the most appropriate structure in memory that will help in processing a new input. When no one episode is that closely related to an input, we can still process it, but no reminding occurs.

One thing that is obvious about reminding is that the more you know about a subject, the more you can be reminded of, within the course of processing inputs related to that subject. Thus, experts in particular fields might be expected to have reminding experiences directly tied in with their expertise. For certain people, we might expect reminding experiences corresponding to:

1. known chess patterns
2. known political patterns
3. previously encountered similar situations
4. patterns of behavior of a particular individual
5. relatedness of scientific theories
6. types of football plays
7. kinds of music or paintings

Why is it that some people are reminded of a famous chess game upon viewing another game and some people are not? The answer, obviously is that not everyone has knowledge of famous chess games. Obvious as this may be, it says something very important about memory: We use what we know to help us process what we receive. We would be quite surprised if a chess expert were *not* reminded of a famous chess game upon seeing one just like it. We expect an expert to have categorized his experiences in such a way as to have them available for aid in processing new experiences. (An interesting problem here is that people can be reminded of something on occasion but can fail to evoke the same memory in a similar circumstance. This is a property of a dynamic memory, its changeability makes people's memory systems function differently in apparently similar situations.)

Thus, reminding is not a phenomenon that just happens to occur to some people at some times. It is a phenomenon that must occur, that as human understanders we expect to occur, in an individual who has a certain set of knowledge organized in a fashion that is likely to bring that knowledge to bear at a certain time.

This implies that an expert is constantly receiving new inputs and evaluating them and understanding them in terms of previously processed inputs. We understand in terms of what we already understood. But, trite as this may seem, this view of understanding has not been seriously pursued either by psychologists interested in understanding or by Artificial Intelligence (AI) researchers interested in understanding or in expert systems. To build an expert system, two possible avenues are open. One is to attempt to get at the compiled knowledge of the expert; that is, the rules he uses when he makes the decisions that reflect his expertise (see Buchanan et al., 1976; Davis, 1976; and Feigenbaum, 1977 for examples of this work). This approach has the advantage of being orderly and methodical. Its disadvantage is that such a system would not be able to reorganize what it knew. It would thus have a difficult time learning.

An alternative is to attempt to model the raw memory of the expert. This would involve creating a set of categories of subdomains of the expertise in question and equipping the system with rules for the automatic modification of those categories. Such a system would attempt to process new experiences in terms of the most closely related old experiences available. Upon finding an episode that strongly related, whatever that might turn out to mean, a reminding would occur. The new episode would then be indexed in terms of the old episode. New categories would be built as needed when old categories turned out to be useless from either under-utilization or over-utilization, or because the expectations contained within them were too often wrong.

An expert then is someone who gets reminded of just the right prior experience to help him in processing his current experiences. But, in a sense, we are all experts. We are experts on our own experiences. We all must utilize some system of categories, and rules for modifying those categories to help us find what we know when we need to know it.

Some things to consider are:

1. What is it that we do to new inputs while processing them that seems to automatically make conscious the most relevant old information?
2. How have prior experiences been categorized or labeled such that they will show up (i.e., be called to mind) at precisely the right moment?

There is one other point to be made here. We are not always reminded of our most relevant prior experience in processing a new input. Thus, another question must also be put:

3. How can we have (mis)classified an experience so as to not bring it to mind at an appropriate time?

So, how do we get reminded? This problem is clearly strongly related to the problem of how we process new inputs at all. If reminding naturally occurs during processing by a dynamic memory system, how we get reminded and how we process ought to amount to different views of the same mechanism.

Let's consider an example of reminding. There is an otherwise ordinary table-service restaurant in Boston, Legal Seafood, where you are asked to pay the check before the food comes. Going to another table-service restaurant where one paid after ordering should normally cause one to be reminded of Legal Seafood if one had been to Legal Seafood. How is such reminding likely to take place?

A script-based view of the processing involved here has the restaurant script being called into play to help process any restaurant experience. In attempting to account for reminding within the natural course of script-based processing, it becomes clear that scripts must be *dynamic memory structures*. That is, given the phenomenon of reminding and what we said above about the relatedness of reminding and processing , a script cannot be a static (that is, unchangeable) data structure. Rather, the restaurant script must actually contain particular memories, such as the experience in Legal Seafood, and must be capable of accumulating new episodes that it has helped to process.

Let's consider this point more carefully. We are arguing that a script is a collection of specific memories organized around common points. Part of the justification for this modification of our old view of scripts is that it really is not possible to say *exactly* what is and what is not part of any script. Particular experiences invade our attempts to make generalizations. To put this another way, we do not believe in the script as a kind of semantic memory data structure, apart from living, breathing, episodic memories. What we know of restaurants is compiled from a multitude of experiences with them, and these experiences are stored with what we have compiled.

A script is built up over time by repeated encounters with a situation. When an event occurs for the first time it is categorized uniquely. (Actually things are rarely seen as being entirely unique.) Repeated encounters with similar events cause an initial category to contain more and more episodes. Elements of those episodes that are identical are treated as a unit, a script. But, subsequent episodes that differ from the script partially are attached to the part of a script that they relate to. The differing parts of the episode are stored in terms of their difference from the script.

In this way, such episodes can be found when similar differences are encountered during processing.

Thus, we want to consider a script as an active memory organizer. It is this view of a script that is relevant in the Legal Seafood example. When we hit a deviation from our normal expectations in a script, and a previously processed episode is relevant to that deviation, we can expect to be reminded of that episode, so that that entire episode can help us in processing the current experience.

One thing that we are arguing against here is the notion of a track that we put forth previously (Schank & Abelson, 1977). A track was a script-like substructure that in form was just like any other script piece. It was called into play when some deviation from the norm was encountered. But, what really seems to happen is that, rather than finding new script pieces to help us when our expectations foul up, we find actual, real live memories. We then use these memories to help us in processing. That is, we formulate new expectations from these experiences that help us to understand our new experience in terms of the relevant old one that has been found.

Thus we are arguing that scripts actually have a stronger role than we had previously supposed. One of their primary functions is as organizers of information in memory. The restaurant script, for example, organizes various restaurant experiences such that when a deviation from the normal flow of the script occurs, the most relevant experience (the one that has been indexed in terms of that deviation) comes to mind. It comes to mind so that expectations can be derived from it about what will happen next in the new experience. Thus, reminding, in a sense, forces us to make use of prior knowledge to form expectations.

One important consequence of the reminding phenomenon is that it alters our view of what it means to understand. For example, when we enter Burger King, having before been to McDonald's but never having been to Burger King, we are confronted with a new situation which we must attempt to *understand*. We can say that a person understands such an experience (i.e., he understands Burger King in the sense of being able to operate in it) when he says "Oh I see, Burger King is just like McDonald's," and then begins to use his information about McDonald's to help him in processing what he encounters at Burger King.

To put this another way, we might expect that at some point during a trip to eat at a Burger King, a person might be *reminded* of McDonald's. Understanding means being reminded of the closest previously experienced phenomenon. That is, when we are reminded of some event or experience in the course of undergoing a different experience, this reminding behavior is not random. We are reminded of a particular experience because the structures we are using to process the new experience are the same structures we are using to organize memory. We cannot help but pass through the old memories while processing a new input.

Finding the *right* one (that is, the one that is most specific to the experience at hand) is what we mean by understanding. Does this mean that episodic memory structures and processing structures are the same thing? The answer is yes. It follows then that there is no permanent (i.e., unchangeable) data structure in memory that exists solely for processing purposes. Scripts, plans, goals, and any other structures that are of use in understanding must be useful as organizing storage devices for memories. These structures exist to help us make sense of what we have seen and will see. Thus, memory structures for storage and processing structures for analysis of inputs are exactly the same structures.

According to this view, it is hardly surprising that we are reminded of similar events. Since memory and processing structures are the same, sitting right at the very spot most relevant for processing will be the experience most like the current one. Thus, the discovery of a coherent set of principles governing what is likely to remind one of what is a crucial step, not only in research on the organization of memory, but also for natural language processing in general. We will now consider reminding in more detail.

Types of reminding

The word *remind* is used in English to mean a great many different things. Joe can *remind you of* Fred. You can ask someone to *remind you to do something*. We get reminded of a good joke, of past experiences, of things we intended to do and so on.

The type of reminding that we have been discussing is what we call *processing-based reminding*. This is the kind of reminding that occurs during the normal course of understanding or processing some new information as a natural consequence of the processing of that information.

In a broad categorization of reminding, two other types of reminding come up that bear superficial similarity to processing-based reminding, but which are not relevant for our purposes here. The first of these is what we term *dictionary-based reminding*. Often when we look up a word in our *mental dictionaries*, we find an entire episode from our experience located with the definition, almost as if it were a part of that definition. Such dictionary-based reminding clearly cannot occur for words that are in great use in our daily lives. But for words, concepts, or objects that we use infrequently, such reminding is likely to occur. Thus, *Toyota* can bring to mind a particular Toyota and an experience associated with it. Similarly, phrases, such as "I am not a crook," or "I am the greatest," bring to mind particular episodes. Dictionary-based reminding is easily accounted for. Our mental dictionaries do not look like Webster's. Information about how to use a word or phrase, what circumstances it first appeared in for you, who uses it, the classes of things it can be applied to, feelings associated with it, and so on, are part of our mental entry for a word. In a sense, the less that is there, the more we notice it. As we gather a great deal of information about a word, the particular memories that we have associated with it tend to lose their connection to the word. Only the essential user-definition remains.

Thus, dictionary-based reminding is a phenomenon that helps to define a word for us in terms of a particular memory. This is not very useful in the long run. In fact, if we treated every word like that, we would find it very difficult to actually process anything in a reasonable amount of time. Such reminding is an important part of initial concept formation, however. Thus, there is a sense in which when such reminding does not occur, we may well have understood better, since the concept is more universally, that is, less particularly, defined.

Actually, dictionary-based reminding is a processing type of reminding too, namely one having to do with the processing of words (and sometimes objects). But, dictionary-based reminding is not very relevant to the operation of a dynamic episodic memory.

The second kind of reminding that is irrelevant to our discussion here is *visually-based reminding*. Sometimes one thing just looks like another. Since our minds organize perceptual cues and find items in memory based on such cues, it is hardly surprising that such reminding should occur. In processing-based reminding, the best reminding that should occur is the one we are least likely to notice. When we enter a restaurant we have been to before, the order of processing, that is, our expectations about the events in that restaurant, and their subsequent realization, should remind us of that restaurant. In other words, we process to what we perceive to be the closest fitting memory structure. If there is an exact fit, we are processing to the structure that contains the episode that fits. We do not feel that we have been reminded because reminding occurs when the fit is approximate, not exact. Nonetheless, in the strict sense of reminding we have been reminded of exactly the right thing.

The same thing ocurs in perceptual processing. In processing John's face, the best fit is the memory piece that contains the perceptual features for John's face. We do not feel reminded by this, we simply feel that we have recognized the set of perceptual features. We feel reminded there too, when the fit is approximate. A new person can physically remind us of one we already have features in our mind for, because there is a partial match.

It is easy to confuse visually-based reminding with processing-based reminding. Visual processing is a kind of processing of course, so they are quite close. Moreover, frequently, after an approximate perceptual match has been made, an episode from memory comes to mind that is associated with that approximate perceptual match. This is the visual analogue of dictionary-based reminding. Associated with the perceptual features of an object that has not been accessed a great many times will be one or more experiences connected to that object. Once the input has triggered a structure in memory that defines the input, memory is not overly concerned with whether the input was the perception of sights or sounds. However, the kind of reminding that we are interested in is situation-based, not perception-based. That is, in processing a situation, when one is reminded of another situation, the new situation should be quite relevant to our understanding of the original situation.

Types of processing-based reminding

We can now discuss the kinds of processing-based reminding that there are. If we can determine some of the kinds of reminding experiences (from here on, when we say reminding, we shall mean processing-based situational reminding) that there are, then we will have, at the same time, determined some of the possible organizational strategies that there are in memory. Reminding is the result of similar organization, after all. Thus, one can help in the discovery of the other.

Reminding based upon event expectations

The first type of reminding that we shall discuss is the kind we were referring to the Legal Seafood example. This reminding is based on the assumptions about processing that were captured by the notion of scripts as presented in Schank and Abelson (1977). (The definition of a script that we shall use in this book is considerably more restricted than our old definition. But, the particulars of wht is and is not a script need not concern us at this point. We shall return to this issue in Chapter 5.)

The assumption that is relevant is that, given an action, it is reasonable to expect that another particular action will follow. In other words, it seems to be true that, as processors of the world around us, we make assumptions about what will happen next. Such assumptions are often based upon what we know about the situation we are in.

Whatever structural entities actually have the responsibility for encoding such expectations should serve both as memory organizers and as data structures used in processing. Such structures contain predictions and expectations about the normal flow of events in some standardized situation.

In such a structure, whenever an expectation derived from that structure fails, its failure is marked. Thus, any deviation from the normal flow of events, in a structure whose task it is to encode expectations about the normal flow of events, is remembered by indexing that structure with a pointer to the episode that caused the expectation failure. That index is placed at the point of deviation. Thus, if ordering in a restaurant is handled by expectations derived from a restaurant structure, then the Legal Seafood experience would cause an expectation failure in that structure. In that case, the Legal Seafood experience would be stored in memory in terms of a failed expectation about ordering in a standard restaurant.

Thus, reminding that is based upon expectations about events occurs when the structure that was directing processing produces an expectation that does not work the way it was supposed to. This kind of reminding occurs whenever a deviation occurs in the normal flow of events in a structure. At the end of these deviations are indices that characterize the nature of the deviation. A match on the index brings to light the memory stored there.

Consider a script we might call **ride in airplane.** Under the event of serving drinks we might find memories about **drinks spilled on lap, free drinks, drunken party in next seat,** and so on. Each of these are potential indices, based on expectation failures from one's own experience, under which actual memories are found.

We would expect then, that all of one's experiences inside an airplane are organized by some airplane structure (as well as by other structures that might also be relevant). These particular memories are indexed according to their peculiar attributes with respect to the event in the relevant script piece.

According to this view there are two key questions:

1.   What are the categories or classes of memory structures?
2.   How are indices formed and used in memory organization within a structure?

In addition there is a third question. Not all reminding is neatly restricted within a given memory structure that reflects one particular context (such as restaurants and airplanes). Sometimes reminding can occur across such structures. Thus we have the question:

1. How does a memory organized in one memory structure remind you of something that would naturally be classed in a different structure?

The answer to this last question is a key problem before us in this book. It is important to understand why it is a key question within the bounds of processing-based reminding.

Recall that in studying processing-based reminding we are trying to discover how an extremely relevant memory can be brought to the fore in the natural course of processing. In the kind of reminding we just discussed, we suggested that one way such reminding occurs is this: In attempting to make predictions about what will happen next in a sequence of events, a relevant structure is brought in. In the course of applying the expectations derived from that structure, we attempt to get the most specific expectations to apply. Often these must be found by using an actual memory which has been stored under a failure of one of the expectations that is part of that structure. Thus, to get reminded in this way, there must have been an initial match on the basis of an identity between the structure now active and the one originally used to process the recalled episode (i.e. the one you were reminded of).

Now, the question is, can we ever get reminded of something that is not from a close match in an identical structure? It is obvious that people do get reminded across contextually-bounded structures of the type we have been using for illustration here. That is, a reminded event can have something in common with the initial event, but that common element does not have to be its physical or societal situation. But how can such reminding occur, if all memories are stored in terms of structures such as the scripts of Schank and Abelson (1977)?

It is obvious that it cannot. As we said in that book, many different types of structures govern processing. We made distinctions between plan application, goal tracking, and script application, often seeming to suggest that the *correct level of processing* flitted from one to the other. What seems clear now is that memories are stored at all levels and that processing of inputs must take place on each level.

That is, at the same time that we are applying a script-like structure, we are also processing the same input in a number of different ways. To find out what those other ways are, we must take a look at other kinds of reminding.

Goal-based reminding

In processing an input we are not only attempting to understand each event that happens as an event itself. We are also attempting to get a larger picture, to see the forest for the trees so to speak. We not only want to know what happened but why it happened. Thus we must track goals.

An example here will serve to illustrate goal-based reminding. Someone told me about an experience of waiting on a long line at the post office and noticing that the person ahead had been waiting all that time to buy one stamp. This reminded me of people who buy a dollar or two of gas in a gas station.

What could be the connection? One possibility is that I had characterized such motorists as *people who prefer to do annoying tasks over and over when they could have done them less often if they had purchased larger quantities in the first place.* Now such a category is extremely bizarre. That is, it is unlikely that there is such a structure in memory. The existence of so complex a structure would imply that we are simply creating and matching categories in our heads in order to be reminded. As this seems rather unreasonable, we must look for some more realistic way of explaining such a reminding.

Recall that processing considerations are intimately connected with memory categorizations. If we ask what kind of processing issues might be in common between the post office experience and the gas station experience, we find that in the *goal-based* analysis of the kind we have proposed in Schank and Abelson (1977), there is a very obvious similarity here. Both stories related to goal subsumption failures (Wilensky, 1978). In processing any story we are trying to find out why the actor did what he did. Questions about the motivations of an actor are made and answered until a level of goal-based or theme-based explanation is reached. In this story, why the person bought a stamp is easy, as is why he stood in line. But good goal-based processing should note that this story is without point if only those two goals are tracked (Schank & Wilensky, 1977). The *point* of the story is that the actor's behavior was somehow unusual. This unusualness was his failure to think about the future. In particular, he could have saved himself future effort by buying more stamps either before now or at this time. But he failed to *subsume* this goal. Thus the story is telling us about a goal-subsumption failure of a particular kind. Understanding this story involves understanding the kind of goal-subsumption failure that occurred.

Thus there are a set of memories organized by *goal-subsumption fail-*

ures in much the same way as script-like structures organized memories earlier. Here too, there are a set of indices on particular kinds of goal-subsumption failures. One of these has to do with waiting in line for service. That is where the gas station experience sits in memory. The new post office experience is processed using structures that track goals. At the same time it is being processed using structures that carry expectations based upon particular contexts. As it happens there are no relevant processing predictions that come from the script-like structures here. The contexts in the reminding are quite different. But the goal tracking causes a reminding that can have potentially useful consequences if it is desirable to attempt to understand the motivations of the actor in the events that were described. Our assertion is that, as processors we always seek an understanding of why people do what they do. Reminding that occurs in response to our questioning ourselves about why an actor did what he did can be useful for making significant generalizations (i.e., learning). In other words, attempting to understand at the level of goals can lead to a generalization that may be valid in future processing.

Consider another example of goal-based reminding. Recently my secretary took a day off because her grandmother died. My previous secretary had had a great many relatives die and was gone a great deal because of it. It is not surprising that one experience reminded me of the other. Furthermore, I could not help but make predictions based upon the first secretary's subsequent behavior with respect to the second's future behavior. Consciously, I knew that these predictions were useless since there was no similarity between the two people, but the reminding occurred nevertheless.

What could a memory structure be like in which both these experiences would be stored? Again, we do not want to have static nodes in memory such as *employee's relative dies* (the hierarchical superset in both cases). Our memory connections must have processing relevance which may or may not be semantic superset relevance. (In this example, I had had other employee's relatives dies, but I was not reminded of those experiences.)

Here again goal-tracking causes a recognition that goal subsumption failure has occurred. One method of goal subsumption is to hire a secretary. I had processed both of these situations with respect to how they related to him. They both caused a particular goal-subsumption of mine (the same one) to be temporarily blocked. The temporary blocking of secretarial work due to the death of a relative is an index under goal-subsumption failure. The reminding that occurred, again had the possibility of applying what occurred in the first situation to the understanding of the second. In this instance, that application was deemed to be irrelevant by X. But the recognition of like patterns from which generalizations (and thus predictions about the future) can be made, is very important for a knowing system. The fact that the particular reminding was of no use here does not obviate the general significance of such goal-based remindings.

One key issue in the reminding and memory storage problem, then, is the question of what higher level memory structures are used in processing a new input. We have already worked with some of these structures in Schank and Abelson (1977), Wilensky (1978), and Carbonell (1979). We have recognized such structures as Goal-Blockage, Goal-Failure, Goal-Replacement, and Goal-Competition, not to mention the various structures associated with satisfying a goal. Each time one of these goal-based structures is accessed during normal processing, that structure becomes a source of predictions that are useful for future processing and learning via reminding. Structures based upon goal-tracking are thus likely to be of significance in a memory that can get reminded.

Plan-based reminding

It follows that if goals are being tracked, then so are the plans that are created to satisfy these goals. If we are to learn from our remindings, and that does seem to be one of the principal uses of reminding, then we must learn at every level for which we have knowledge. It follows then, that there should be a reminding that is plan-based. Such remindings should facilitate our construction of better plans.

Consider the following example. Recently my daughter was diving in the ocean looking for sand dollars. I pointed out where a group of them were, yet she proceeded to dive elsewhere. I asked why and she told me that the water was shallower where she was diving. This reminded me of the old joke about the drunk searching for his lost ring under the lamppost where the light was better.

People quite commonly undergo such reminding experiences, jokes or funny stories being common types of things to be reminded of. What types of processing does such a reminding imply?

The implication is that, just as script-like structures must be full of indices to particular episodes that either justify various expectations or that codify past failed expectations, so are plans used as a memory structures as well. How would this work in this case? Here, the similarity in these two stories is that they both employed some plan that embodied the idea of *looking where it is convenient.* But it is not the plan itself that is the index here. One could correctly pursue that plan and not be reminded of the drunk and the lamppost. The reminding occurs because this plan has occurred in a context where that plan should have been known by the planner to be a bad plan. We shall discuss the difficulties involved in this example and what they imply later on. For now, the main point is that memories are stored in terms of plans too. Hence, reminding can also be plan-based.

Reminding across multiple contexts

There is no reason why reminding must be limited to the kinds of structures and processing that we have previously worked on, and indeed it is not. Reminding can take place in terms of high level structural patterns that cut across a sequence of events, as opposed to the reminding that we have been discussing thus far – reminding that occurs at particular points in the processing of individual events. This kind of reminding occurs when a pattern of events, as analyzed in broad, goal-related terms, is detected and found to be similar to a previously perceived pattern from another context.

To consider an example: We can imagine a head of state on a state visit getting into an argument that disrupts the visit. Hearing about this could remind you of arguments with your mother on a visit. It could also remind you of a rainstorm during a picnic. Recall that any given input is processed on many different levels simultaneously. Imagine a context in which our supposed head of state visit took a great deal of planning, went smoothly at the outset, was expected to have great ramifications for future efforts at consummating an important deal, and then went awry because of some capricious act under the control of no one in particular that caused the argument and the subsequent diplomatic rift. The same sort of thing could be happening at a well-planned picnic that was intended to have important personal or business ramifications and then got fouled up because of the weather that in turn permanently ruined the pending deal.

A less fanciful example of the same phenomenon occurs in watching a play or movie. If you have seen *Romeo and Juliet* and are watching *West Side Story* for the first time, it is highly likely that at some point in the middle of *West Side Story* you will notice that it is the *Romeo and Juliet* story in a modern-day New York, with music. Such a realization is a reminding experience of the classic kind. That is, this reminding represents true understanding of the kind we mentioned earlier between McDonald's and Burger King. Here again the reminding matches the most relevant piece of memory and that brings with it a great many expectations that are both relevant and valid.

But the complexity in matching *West Side Story* to *Romeo and Juliet* is tremendous. In the Burger King example, it was only necessary to be in some sort of **fast food** script and proceed merrily down that script. But in this example, everything is superficially different. The city is New York, there is a gang warfare, there are songs. To see *West Side Story* as an instance of *Romeo and Juliet* one must be not only processing the normal complement of scripts and goals. One must also be, in a sense, summarizing the overall plot to oneself, because that is where the match occurs.

Thus, we have yet another level of analysis that people must be engaged in, in understanding, that of making an overall assessment of events in terms of their goals, the conditions that obtain during the pursuit of those goals, the events of their actions, the interpersonal relationships that are affected, and the eventual outcome of the entire situation.

Morals

When a new input is received, in addition to all the other analyses we have suggested, we also tend to draw conclusions from what we have just processed. Often these conclusions themselves can remind us of something. A moral derived from a story, the realization of the *point* of the story, and so on, can each serve as an index to memories that have been stored in terms of the points they illustrate or the messages they convey.

Such reminding depends, of course, on our having made the actual categorization or index for the prototypical story. In other words, unlike the other kinds of reminding that we have so far discussed, here we would have had to pre-analyze the prototypical story in terms of its moral message or point. Indeed, we probably do just that. Why else would we choose to remember a joke or story unless it had a point we were particularly fond of?

But here the problem is one of finding the adage or joke that is relevant. We found the *drunk* joke mentioned earlier because the plans being used were the same. Similarly, we can find morals when physical or situational structures such as scripts are the same. But what do we do when the only similarity is the moral itself? To find memories that way implies that there are higher level structures in memory that correspond to such morals. This also involves being reminded across contexts. We shall have to come up with structures that can account for such remindings.

Intentional reminding

The last type of reminding we shall discuss is what we label intentional reminding. Sometimes one can get reminded of something by just the right mix of ingredients, by the right question to memory, so to speak. In those circustances, reminding is not directly caused by the kind of processing that we are doing at the time. Rather, the processing is directed by the desire to call a relevant past experience to mind. It is as if we were trying to be reminded. We, as processors, know that if only we were to be reminded of something here, it would help us in our processing. We thus try to get reminded. If we are trying to answer a question, then reminding is a form of getting the answer. In other words, we try to remind ourselves of the answer. But, even if what we are doing is simply trying to understand a situation, intentional reminding represents our attempt to come up with a relevant experience that will help us to understand our current situation. Not all intentional reminding is consciously intended, however. Much of it comes from just thinking about what is happening to us at a given time, without any conscious feeling that we wish we were reminded of something. Our thinking of a way to solve a particular problem often causes us to be reminded.

On a walk on the beach, I was asked by the person whom I was walking with if he should take his dog along. This reminded me of the last time I had been visiting someone and had gone for a walk and had taken the resident dog along. I had objected, but my host said that we had to take it, and with good reason (protecting us from other dogs), it turned out. This reminding experience caused me to ask myself if we would *need* the dog on the beach in the same way. I thought not and said so.

The above is an example of intentional reminding. Had I not been reminded at all, I would have simply responded that I didn't want to take the dog, since I don't especially like dogs. Instead I posed a problem to myself. Knowing how and when to pose that problem (here, finding the possible advantages of taking the dog) is a complex problem which is discussed in Chapter 4 and in Schank (1981). To solve this problem, I attempted to be reminded of a relevant experience, if there was one.

Intentional reminding is extremely common. It forms the basis of a good deal of our conversation and of our thought. We try to get reminded by narrowing the contexts that we are thinking about until a memory item is reached. This narrowing is effected by a series of indices. Often these indices are provided by the input, but sometimes they must be provided by the person doing the thinking in an attempt to consciously narrow the context.

In the situation above, two contexts were active: *visiting a colleague at his home* and *taking a walk*. Each of these contexts alone had too many experiences in it to come up with any actual memories. But the index of *dog* changes things. The *dog* index is what is necessary to focus the search. Here *taking the dog* was a sufficient cue for me because I so rarely did it.

The process of searching memory depends upon having a set of structures that adequately describe the contents of memory and a set of indices that point out the unusual features of the structures. Given such entities, it is then possible to search memory for intentional reminding.

As another example, my wife referred to the fact that we had eaten a pineapple in Hawaii when we were last there. I couldn't recall it. I asked where we had eaten it. She said the beach. That didn't help. I tried to imagine the beach belonging to the hotel we stayed at, but remembered that it didn't have a beach. I tried to imagine eating a pineapple in other contexts around the hotel in case she was mistaken, but couldn't. Finally I took myself mentally around the island, looking for beaches, that is, setting cues of unique scenes for myself. Finally I found a beach that set up a scene that did have pineapple eating in it (along with a picture of everything else that happened at that beach).

The point here is that memory search is constrained by the organization of memory. In order to search effectively we must attempt to *remind* ourselves of what we are looking for. To do this means locating the memory/processing structure that was used to understand the material being searched for in the first place. This requires *putting yourself* in the original processing situation. That is, if we can get ourselves to process the right kind of input, we can find what we are looking for in memory.

A perspective on reminding

Reminding, then, is a highly significant phenomenon that has much to say to us about the nature of memory. It tells us about how memory is organized. It also tells us about learning and generalization. If memory has within it a set of structures, it seems obvious that these structures cannot be immutable. As new information enters memory, the structures adapt. Adapting initially means storing new episodes in terms of old expectations generated by existing structures. Eventually expectations that used to work will have to be invalidated. Indices that were once useful will cease to be of use because the unique instances they indexed are no longer unique. New structures will have to be built.

Reminding serves as the start of all this. As a result, looking at reminding gives a snapshot of memory at an instant of time. Ater that snapshot has been taken, memory must adjust by somehow combining the old reminded episode with the newly processed episode to form a generalization that will be of future use in processing. Thus, reminding not only tells us about memory organization, it also signals memory that it will have to adapt to the current episode. Reminding is the basis for learning.

3 Failure-driven memory

At the root of our ability to understand is our ability to find the most relevant memory at just the right time. This can mean being able to tell a good story that illustrates a point, as well as being able to recall a prior experience that will shed light on how we should act in a given situation. To bring exactly the right experience to mind at exactly the right time requires a memory organization that is capable of indexing episodes in such a way as to have them available for use when they are needed. This implies an indexing scheme that has at its base processing considerations. That is, if a particular memory is relevant to processing at a certain point, it should ideally be indexed in terms of that relevance. Processing relevance means the ability to come to mind at just the point where that memory would be most useful for processing. This tends to be necessary when things have not gone exactly as planned. That is, when we have failed to predict accurately what will happen next, we are most in need of a specific memory to help us out. One way to do this is to index memories in terms of their relationship to processing prediction failures.

When processing predictions fail, a notation is made with respect to that failure. This notation serves as an index to memories in terms of their future processing relevance, i.e., in special cases that have proved difficult to predict accurately in our prior experience. When a similar failure occurs, the memory that was stored in terms of that failure is retrieved and made available for use. We call this conception of memory failure-driven memory.

Let us consider the notion of how failure-driven memory affects our view of memory structures. For example, consider again how to represent information about restaurants, but this time from the view of a continually evolving, failure-driven, memory.

In Schank and Abelson (1977), we treated every individual restaurant episode as having a pointer to the restaurant script which would help fill in the details upon recall. The advantage of this scheme was to avoid storing uniquely all the parts of a restaurant experience that are invariant across restaurants. Once an episode was identified as being restaurant-related, it was stored rather simply. For example, $RESTAURANT$ (John, Lobster, Lundy's) was what we proposed for an episode that was solely about John eating lobster in Lundy's.

While this scheme is sensible on the surface, it has some underlying problems. It treats everything equally, for one thing. That is, all restaurant experiences would be stored as a unit in terms of the script. Consider two restaurant experiences that are vitually identical except for what was ordered. It would be easy to get confused about aspects of these two experiences, which waitress (if there were two different ones in the same restaurant) served which food, for example. Such confusions are not accounted for in the original scheme where each story is uniquely stored. The structure we used before would have the waitress, the food, the weather, or whatever all stored together in the same unit with a link to the restaurant script. Our computer wouldn't get confused by two similar episodes, but people would: why?

The reason for people's confusion of similar episodes must have to do with the way they store those episodes. It seems likely that similar things are stored in terms of each other, i.e., they are *mushed* together. Unique entities, those that differ from the *standard mush*, are stored in terms of the *mush* with their differences indicated. One restaurant is like another. For the purposes of economy of storage, we need not remember the details of every restaurant we have been to. We can reconstruct that we must have ordered or that we probably sat down from what we know about restaurants. This implies that what we are doing when we store something is checking for the features of that experience that are interestingly unique. We then pay particular attention to those features in the storage scheme we employ. What we do not pay particular attention to is stored in terms of the normative flow of events, that is, the mush of memories which becomes the standard set of script actions, or the backbone of a script.

In order to account for the reminding phenomena we have been discussing, a storage scheme such as the one we are proposing would have to have entire episodes available for reminding at certain points along the backbone of a script. One of the purposes of reminding is to provide relevant predictions at a critical point in processing. A script is also a bundle of relevant predictions. A script must serve as an organizational tool by which episodes that have predictive value in processing can be stored in such a way as to facilitate the retrieval of those episodes at the right point.

Recall that we are looking for an organizational structure that integrates the structures of processing with those of memory. That is, we desire to have episodes stored in such a way that each one of them can serve as a kind of script itself. We want predictions to be available from *all* prior experiences, not just those that we have abstracted as scripts or script pieces. After all, people make predictions about what will happen next based on both particular episodes they have found in memory and generalizations drawn from similar (mushed) experiences. Scripts must do more than simply govern processing by making predictions and filling in causal chain inferences. A person who has experienced something only once will expect his second time around to conform to the intial experience and will be *surprised* in some sense, when the second experience does not conform to the first. Scripts must account for understanding based upon singular instances as well. The reason that this is also the province of scripts is that any unique episode will have been processed by the structure most similar to it. In other words, a script will have been used for a while in processing a unique episode, and then will have been found wanting. Memory is likely to reflect that processing experience.

What we are dealing with here is the script acquisition problem. This is how scripts get put together in the first place: first one experience, then another on top of it, strengthening those areas of agreement and beginning to solidify a script. Obviously there are times when *new* experiences for which there is one or no prior experience can be understood in terms of old ones. That is, such new experiences need not be new in every way. The new parts of an experience can most certainly occur within well trodden contexts. Thus, when you go to Legal Seafood you make a note that, in this instance, it was necessary to modify your restaurant script so as to indicate that the PAYING scene has been placed immediately after the ORDERING scene in memory. The point is, we always try to understand by using our past experience.

We are proposing here that the significant parts of entire episodic memories are stored at critical script junctures. Previously we had codified such junctures as *tracks* of scripts that were themselves script-like in nature. Now we are suggesting that what is stored at the juncture are specific episodes. If similar junctures repeatedly occur, then tracks might get built, but that is not the key point. Memories can be organized by scripts, retrieved by scripts during reconstruction, and found for processing use at just the point where the script-based predictions fail. That is when script-based reminding occurs. Thus, for Legal Seafood, the entire memory experience is available at the point of interruption or abnormality following the ORDERING scene. Or, to put it another way, we recall our entire Legal Seafood experience because it was indexed in terms of the faulty prediction of the ORDERING scene of the restaurant script. We are reminded of that episode when similar failures in prediction occur. We use those episodes to help us process new experiences that cause the same processing failures (i.e. that *remind* us of the same processing failures). This episode is used, just as any script is used, to predict what will happen next and to fill in the causal chain by making inferences.

Deep down inside the guts of a script, we find links to every unique memory experience we have had that has been processed in terms of that script. (These pointers can be obliterated when a previously unique episode recurs. At that point, a new script may be formed that is independent of the original.) Thus script application is embellished by going down paths which the script itself organizes that contain all prior deviant (that is, not completely standard) experiences. These experiences are functionally identical to scripts and thus are integral parts of the application process. This can occur within any script-piece at all.

As an example of all this, consider Figure 1, a picture of a possible set of memory experiences tied to, or organized by, the restaurant script.

This diagram illustrates the use of a script as an organizer of information in memory. The restaurant script that we have used in the past is no more than the standard default path, or basic organizing units, that serve as the backbone for all remembered restaurant experiences that have been stored as restaurant experiences. Every important deviation from the standard script is stored as a modification of the particular scene in which the deviation occurred.

So, one experience in Legal Seafood causes a deviation (these were previously referred to as being on the *weird list* in Schank and Abelson 1977) in the ordering scene. This deviation serves as both the beginning of a reminding experience and part of the script application process (as well as the start of the script acquisition process). As we have been saying, storage and processing must be taken care of by the same mechanisms in order to get natural reminding to take place. In addition, the scheme that we are proposing allows for the use of all prior experiences in the interpretation of new experiences, rather than a reliance solely on standard normalized experiences (i.e., what we have previously called scripts). This scheme works as follows:

Information about a restaurant is processed by the use of the restaurant script as described in Schank and Abelson (1977) and Cullingford (1978). The major difference is that each scene is applied one by one as needed. Thus, the entire script is not brought in at once. As long as the story fits current expectations (based upon the operating stereotype) no devia-

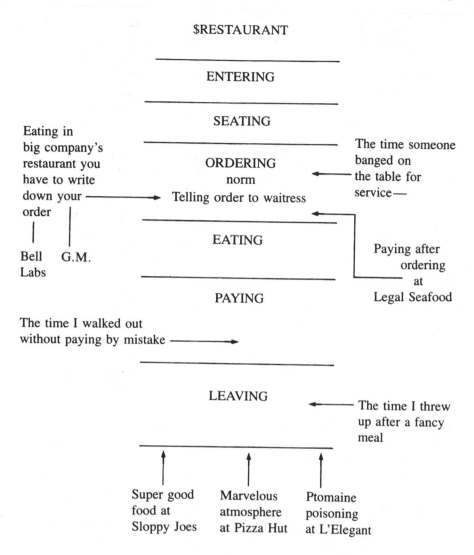

Figure 1

tion from the usual default script is made, and no reminding occurs. Underneath the restaurant script's bare backbone, however, are all the memories that have ever been classified in terms of restaurants. As soon as an abnormal event occurs (i.e., one that is unusual to the extent that its occurrence is not predicted by, or is actually contradicted by, the normal flow of the script), normal processing stops. At this point, an index must be constructed in terms of which the new episode will be stored. Constructing the index is complicated. It depends on finding an explanation for what went wrong in the expectation derived from a scene in the script. This will be seen in the cases discussed later on in this chapter.

In the diagram above, we have four deviations recorded in the ordering scene. In one, there is the experience in which someone at my table banged the silverware on his plate repeatedly to get service. In another, we have the memory of having to write down my order at Bell Labs. We also have a similar experience at General Motors Labs. And, we have the experience in Legal Seafood of being asked to pay immediately after ordering.

The index that points to these experiences as deviations from normal ordering is not a *track* or *subscene* that gives alternative paths through the script. Rather, the entire experience inside the scene that contained the failed expectation is pointed to and recalled. This scene, as it happens, also points to other scenes with which it was associated. Thus, the entire experience at G.M. can be brought to mind if need be. At Bell Labs, I was reminded of G.M. when I was asked to order my food by writing down what I wanted and handing the order to the waitress. I was initially reminded solely of the ordering scene at G.M, but as memory is reconstructive, the ordering scene at G.M. brought to mind the existence of other scenes that occurred that day. These scenes then also became available for my consideration for their possible processing relevance. The recognition of the existence of these other scenes has two possible uses.

First, relevant predictions, of the kind we have previously said were available from scripts, actually come from whatever prior experience is available. Thus, the rest of the happenings at G.M. can then be used to interpret what happens at Bell Labs. Such predictions can even encompass events that are in no way restaurant related. The importance of this capability cannot be overemphasized. *People interpret new experiences in terms of old ones.* The only way to get the relevant older experience to be available is to have been reminded of it in the normal course of processing what was going on in the new experience. Noticing that Bell Labs is like G.M. in the ordering scene can then allow for remembrances of the G.M. experiences to guide future behavior at Bell Labs. In other words, we can then begin to look for similarities in other areas. Reminding is a catalyst for generalization.

Often, of course, there is no need at all for the remembered experience. Once one is reminded of G.M., one can then ignore this reminding; that is, one can decide that no predictions from one experience are relevant in the new experience and one can return to normal processing by going back to the normal backbone of the script to handle future inputs. Alternatively, it is possible to never return at all to the normal script because its predictions are so standard and therefore inappropriate in a novel setting. Instead, the predictions from the reminded events are used to guide processing.

Whatever choice is made, a new episode has been experienced and part of a processor's decisions at this point includes the problem of storing the new episode. First, where are links made to the Bell Labs experience? Second, at what point is the Bell Labs experience broken up into pieces of episodes that lose their relatedness to each other? Third, what is the overall effect on memory and future processing?

The answer to the first question is that since the deviation in ordering has been seen before, a pointer to the G.M. episode that existed previously at the **write down order** deviation is now joined by a pointer to that experience at Bell Labs.

With respect to the second question, we are assuming that a processor would have analyzed the new Bell Labs episodes in terms of all the relevant higher level knowledge structures that were used to process it in the first place. We can expect that structures containing knowledge about *lecturing, talking with colleagues, consulting* and so on, might all have been used in addition to a knowledge structure about restaurants. Some overall structure, such as *visit to a company to lecture* might well exist in the mind of someone who has frequently had such experiences. Thus, it might be possible to find memories contained in each individual structure during a reconstructuve process that utilized a higher level structure that connected them all together. As we shall see later on, these high level structures cannot be immutable across people as long as their role is to reflect (the differing) experiences that people have. Ordinarily then, we would expect that each of these individual structures is not directly connected to any of the others. So our new pointer at the ordering deviation points to the part of the experience that contains **restaurant** and as many other pieces of that experience that may be causally connected to the restaurant part of the entire Bell Labs episode. Other parts of the Bell Labs experience would be stored in terms of the knowledge structures (such as scripts) that processed those parts. Thus, the entire experience is broken up into smaller pieces for processing and storage. It can all be put back together again, if appropriate high level structures exist that contain information about what structures ordinarily link to what other structures. This issue will be discussed in Section III.

We asked about the overall effect on memory of an experience that deviates from the norm. Memory can be affected by such a deviant experience in two possible ways. First, if the deviant experience has no counterpart, e.g., if there had been no prior G.M. experience or if the Bell Labs experience differed at the ordering scene in some significant way from the G.M. experience, then a new deviant path off of the ordering scene (in the first instance) or off of the G.M. deviation (in the second) would have to be created. This deviation would point to the relevant experience at Bell Labs with respect to ordering and would now serve as a new source of relevant predictions if that deviation were encountered again inside the restaurant script. All prior experiences, if classified initially as being interestingly deviant, serve as embellishments to the script of which they are a part and thus as a source of predictions.

If the new experience does have a counterpart, that is, if similar deviations have been met before, at some point these experiences are collected together to form a new structure whose predictions, like the higher level restaurant script itself, are disembodied from actual episodes. Thus, at some point the understander notices that not only the G.M. and Bell Labs restaurants have you write down your own order, but so do various faculty clubs and other company lunchrooms. When enough (probably two is enough but that remains an empirical question) of these are encountered, a new structure will be created such that one will not be reminded of particular experiences that caused the creation of this subscene. As this structure is used, the links to the relevant episodes that helped to create that structure initially, become harder to find. In a sense, the new memory structure is broadened by more experiences at the same time that it is narrowed by the loss of its origins. These origins cannot be remembered in the face of many similar experiences. Thus, an argument at lunch at the Harvard Faculty Club might still be remembered, but it would not be possible to get at it through the deviation in the ordering scene of writing down your order any more than it would be possible to get at it by the sitting down scene or any other scene that was now normalized.

One last possible effect of a deviation from expectation is the abandoning of the original memory structure. Thus, if all restaurants begin to employ the written form of ordering, not only is a new structure created, the original one is seen as a useless structure, which is only of historical interest. Often such abandoned structures reflect views of the world which never were true in the first place, that were simply wrong generalizations from scanty data.

Thus, memory collects similar experiences to make predictions from. Before structures are created that embody generalizations relating to a given situation, remindings of prior experiences serve as the source of relevant knowledge. Uniqueness of experience, or perhaps more accurately, unique classifications of experience, serve as a rich source of understandings about new experiences. Repeated experiences tend to dull a person's ability to respond to the world around him by lulling him to sleep during processing, as it were. One problem here is knowing what items that are unique in an experience are also interesting and potentially relevant later on. Mushing two episodes tends to eliminate their differences. An intelligent processor must be careful not to eliminate interesting differences, nor to especially note dull ones.

Using expectation failures

We now must ask ourselves what general principles there are in all this. How does it happen that we store some memories at deviation points in scripts? Is there something going on here that relates to the other kinds of reminding that we discussed, or is this phenomenon specific to script-based reminding?

From our look at reminding, it would seem that the primary advantage of reminding is its production of a maximally relevant memory for use in making predictions and generalizations. Such predictions can then be used in processing the current episode. Any generalizations that are made can be used to process future episodes that share something in common with the current episode and the reminded episode.

A script is a generalization. A script is a structure with an implicit built-in assumption, namely, that because something has happened many times in a similar way, one should expect that thing to happen in the same way next time. When we are reminded of a memory at a juncture in a script, we are prepared to make another generalization. We can formulate a new script piece, based upon whatever identity we can find in the two memories that have in common their placement at the same juncture in the script. For Legal Seafood, this might be, *restaurants that make you sit at long tables also make you pay after ordering.* Clearly some future encounter would remove this generalization from memory as invalid, but the point here is that we do entertain such hypotheses. When they stand up over time, we have learned a new script or piece of a script.

We can say that reminding is the basis for learning, at least as far as scripts are concerned, but is there something more significant going on?

Stepping back to look at what is going on in script-based reminding, we can see that there is a general notion that pervades the various kinds of reminding that we discussed in Chapter 2, namely, in each of these remindings there was a processing failure of some kind. We made a prediction about what would happen ne*t, and our predictions turned out to be wrong. At the point that we recognized that there was a prediction failure, we were reminded of a similar prediction failure.

We want to argue that memory is failure-driven. We expect our predictions about other people's behavior and processes to be accurate. When they are not, we make note of our error so that we can make better predictions when we encounter the same situation next time. This *notation* has the form of a link to the failure from the episode which caused the failure, indexed in terms of the reason for failure. This is what happened in the script-based remindings above, and it is far more ubiquitous than that.

Lehnert (1979) developed a theory that questions were often best answered by following a trace of the previous processing that had occurred. Thus, in answering a question about a story, one would have to have saved some of the false starts and failed expectations used in processing that story. Some questions would be answered on the basis of those failed expectations. (Granger, 1980, also did some work on this.)

The theory we are proposing is similar in spirit to Lehnert's proposal. We are suggesting that all of memory conforms to her view of question-answering in story processing. We attempt to make predictions about what will happen in any episode we are attempting to comprehend. When we detect a failure of an action to conform to our expectations, we remember that failure. In a sense, we are attempting to jot it down for next time, so that we won't fail that way again and so that we learn from our failures.

Viewed this way, reminding can be seen to be occurring when an expectation is made, but fails to materialize, or, when something happens that was not expected and then happens. Indexed under either of these two kinds of failures are prior failures of the same kind. We get reminded when we notice that we have failed in this way before. From this consistency of failure of the same type, we learn to create better expectations.

Of course not all remindings are of this type, but failure-driven remindings are common enough, and significant enough, to cause us to view memory from that perspective. Clearly, a memory that does not account for such remindings will be of little value in learning and generalization.

Kinds of failures

What kinds of failures in processing expectations can there be? Clearly we have a great many low-level processing expectations, from syntax, phonology, vision, and so on that can fail. Episodic memories are not necessarily indexed off all types of these failures. What we are looking for here are failures of predicted actions on the part of other people, or the world in general.

A large part of what we do in understanding is attempt to predict other people's behavior. We want to understand why someone does something and what he will do next. When we fail in our predictions, we remember our failure for next time. Failure-driven reminding is based in failures in our prediction of other people's action.

To see the kinds of remindings we are talking about, and the way memory is required to deal with them, consider the following reminding experiences (one of which was discussed briefly earlier). (These and other experiences shown here were collected by simply asking colleagues to report remindings that they had.)

A. *The steak and the haircut*
X described how his wife would never make his steak as rare as he liked it. When this was told to Y, it reminded Y of a time, 30 years earlier, when he tried to get his hair cut in a short style in England, and the barber would not cut it as short as he wanted it.

B. *Asking for help*
X was talking about how Y never seemed to ask for help even when it was appropriate to do so. This reminded X of how he had been told that when he ran out of gas in England and asked people in a pub for help, he had violated the rules of behavior in England. Asking for help there was deemed inappropriate, although the person who had told this to X had conceded it was the best plan.

C. *The walking aunt*
X and his family went to a breakfast that was normally held at a school, but this year was held further away. The family had previously walked home from the school, but it was now too far. X's aunt asked to be dropped off at the school after the breakfast so she could walk home as she had done before. This reminded X of a joke about how mathematicians solve problems by reverting to previously solved problems, even if there is a new solution that is simpler than the old.

D. *The sand dollars and the drunk*
X's daughter was diving for sand dollars. X pointed out where there were a great many sand dollars, but X's daughter continued to dive where she was. X asked why. She said that water was shallower where she was diving. This reminded X of the joke about the drunk who was searching for his ring under the lamppost because the light was better there even though he had lost the ring elsewhere.

What do these reminding experiences have in common? They are all examples of a person's inability to correctly predict someone else's behavior. The fact that C and D caused the subject to be reminded of a joke tells us something about jokes as well as about reminding. Jokes are frequently about people's unexpected behavior. To access them in our memories we must have indexed them by their particular type of failures. We retrieve them again when we encounter a similar kind of failure.

Thus a large part of the problem of reminding can be explained by attempting to assess the kinds of failures there are in expectations about other people's behavior. These failures seem to serve as indices to memories. The question is *how?* Consider the kinds of failures exemplified by these cases: In A, we have a failure of a person in a serving role to do what he was asked. In B, we have a failure to act in one's own best interest in the initial episode. The reminding is of someone's suggestion that X *should have* failed to act in his own best interest. In C, we have a failure to produce the best plan for a situation. In D we have the same kind of failure.

Reminding is not so simple a phenomenon that the only identity that exists in these examples is based upon failures. Actually, each of them has in common a number of other features as well. For example, D isn't just a failure to plan optimally. There is also the commonality of searching for something.

Remindings of this sort suggest a view of memory that involves our processing an episode on many levels at once. Essentially, we can view an understanding system as tracking the goals, plans, themes, and other high level knowledge structures that are active in any situation. It is the understander's job to produce sets of expectations about what will happen next at each level of processing. Thus, we have expectations about what the next action to achieve a step in a plan should be, what the next plan to achieve a goal should be, what the next goal in a thematic relation should be, and so on.

Explanations

One of the most interesting facets of human beings is their desire to explain the mysterious. We want to know why a strange thing happened. We want to know why people do what they do. We are unhappy if a person pursues a set of goals that we find incomprehensible, and, when a person fails to do what we expected him to do, we attempt to explain it.

Thus, when our view of what should have happened next in a given situation is found to contradict the facts of the matter, we attempt to *explain* it.

In general we are satisfied with simple explanations; the less work they cause us the better. One of the simplest kinds of explanations is a script. We need only understand that a person is doing what he is doing because he is following a script for us to feel comfortable with having explained his behavior. We can, of course, look for an explanation that is deeper than a script-based one, but we are usually content not to. Thus, an explanation of why one takes off one's shoes in a Japanese restaurant, or why religious Jews always have their head covered, can be answered by *because that's the way it is done in their culture.* Surely there may exist better explanations, for example, because the Japanese sit and sleep on the floor they are more fastidious about its cleanliness; or that Jews come from the desert where head coverings prevent sunstroke. Often the participants in these rituals (or scripts) do not themselves know or believe such explanations. People are usually content with script-based explanations when they are available.

Such explanations are not always available. In the case where no script is in operation, we look for explanations at the level of goals. To explain why someone is doing something, we need to know what goal he is pursuing. This will explain his actions, but only partially. Understanding someone's goal does not always explain his choice of plan to carry out that goal. His choice of a plan may seem very strange indeed, even if we are perfectly cognizant of his goal. For example, we can understand someone wanting to be department chairman, but poisoning the current chairman may seem an odd plan to achieve the goal. So, we also look for explanations at the level of plan choice.

The same is true of goal choice. Sometimes a goal needs to be explained. We may not have any idea why someone would want to be department chairman. In such a case, we look for thematic explanations. That is, we seek to explain goals in terms of higher level goals or themes that obtain for this particular individual. If our department chairman wants the job to please his mother, or to get administrative experiences to help him in a future career, then we are satisfied to some extent by the explanation.

Thus, at the root of our understanding ability is our ability to seek and create explanations. Explanations of human behavior are always grounded in the beliefs of the person we are trying to understand. That is, what we are trying to do when we seek an explanation for an actor's behavior is to find a set of beliefs that the actor could hold that would be consistent with the actions he performed.

Thus, the problem is one of beliefs. Explaining another person's actions requires us to try to *take a look inside his head.* Now consider some possible explanations in the above cases:

A. *The steak and the haircut*
Explanation: The server must believe that X doesn't really want the extreme of what he asked for.

B. *Asking for help*
Explanation: Y and Z must believe that there can be a good reason not to ask for help even if it is the best plan available.

C. *The walking aunt*
Explanation: The planner must believe that to accomplish a goal the best plan is to revert to a previous plan that has worked.

D. *The sand dollars and the drunk*
Explanation: The planner must believe that the easiest plan is the best plan regardless of information to the contrary.

How carefully we examine what other people might believe depends on our need to know. This often reflects our estimates of our future predictive needs. Thus, in Legal Seafood, we can seek an explanation for the actions of the waitress. Her actions are easily explained as *doing what she was told to do because it is her job*. We must then seek an explanation for the behavior of the management of the restaurant, as embodied by the waitress asking for payment at an odd time. Doing this may require us to examine the history of the beliefs of the management, but our need to know is not that great. We are satisfied with an explanation that is script-based because we are not greatly outraged at what has happened in place of what we expected. "That's the way they do it here" will do in cases where we are willing to put up with the inconvenience. We need only mark our script so that we will be able to predict this next time and go on to worry about something else. Of course, if the waitress's aberrant behavior had been to hit us for leaving a poor tip, "that's the way they do it here" would have failed to suffice as an explanation.

The explanation of unexpected behavior by one's friends and acquaintances, and the explanation of odd situations that are important to us, requires more careful attention than attribution to script-based explanations will show. When we fail to predict accurately in those circumstances, we may well want to assess the beliefs of the actor who failed to conform to our expectations. Often such assessments crucially affect our relationship with these people. We might not wish to hang around someone who is willing to kill to get what he wants, for example, or we might want to provide him with a less drastic plan if we are in sympathy with his goal but not his method. Doing this, however, requires us to have correctly assessed his underlying beliefs. Thus, at the root of our ability to operate in the world is our ability to explain the behavior of others by examining their beliefs. (We do explain by examining other aspects of a situation as well. Thus, an explanation that someone was tired, drunk, or stupid will also suffice. In these cases, a processor tends to modify what he knows about a given individual rather than what he knows about a given situation.)

Thus, we are suggesting that indices to memory, and hence our memory organization, are belief-based. The four explanations for the remindings given above are grounded in X's view of what Y believes. The idea here is that we always attempt to explain an actor's behavior. Usually, we have pre-satisfied our need for an explanation by simply noting that the actor did what we expected him to do. When he did not, we must examine the possible belief structures that he may have had at the point of the expectation-failure.

This suggests an algorithm that has the following gross characteristics:

> Utilize the appropriate high level knowledge structure to process input (i.e., scripts, plans, etc.).
> When an expectation generated by those structures fails, attempt to explain the failure.
> To explain a failure of another person to act according to your predictions, attempt to figure out his beliefs. This entails:
> Assessing the implicit beliefs that you expect that person to hold in that situation.
> Producing an Alternative Belief that would be consistent with his behavior.
> Use the Alternative Belief as an index to memory to find other memories previously classified with that Alternative Belief.
> Use other features of the situation as additional indices within the range of behavior delimited by the Alternative Belief to find an actual memory to be used for generalization and modification of predictions.

Thus, what we are proposing here is that memory is organized, at least in part, by a classification of explanations of other people's behavior based upon our assumption of what it is that they must believe. Within that classification, memories from other, quite different, contexts can be found. These memories are indexed by the explanations. A memory is found by noting an expectation failure, deciding upon an explanation, and having decided upon one, noting that a similar explanation has been used before. Explanations are thus somewhat like keys to locked doors. Finding the right key opens the door to reveal a memory.

The key point then is that memory is organized in terms of explanations that we create to help us understand what we receive as input that differs from what we expected.

Now consider one of the above cases viewed from this perspective:

A. *The steak and the haircut:*

1. *Process with knowledge structure.* The first problem in any understanding situation is to find the relevant higher level knowledge structure (such

as a script) to use for processing. Since we are arguing that memories are
stored in terms of prediction failures, and that predictions are made by
higher level knowledge structures, clearly the decision about what
knowledge structure to begin to use in processing is crucial. However, we
also are arguing that processing, and therefore predictions, take place at
many levels at once. Thus, the problem of what knowledge structure to
use in processing is only a problem of which one to use for each level of
processing. That is, we must decide what scripts, plans, goals, and other
structures are applicable. In Section III we will introduce a system of high
level knowledge structures that is more general than that used in Schank
and Abelson (1977). Thus, we shall delay any discussion here of the
problem of selecting a processing structure.

Since the structures we propose in Section III are more general than we
have used previously, for the purposes of this example, we shall just
assume a structure which we shall term PROVIDE-SERVICE. We shall
discuss the validity of such a structure later on.

The assumption here then is that we have recognized, in processing
the story told above about the rare steak, that some structure such as
PROVIDER-SERVICE will be a relevant source of predictions about
why, how, and when a person in a serving role will provide service. This
structure thus provides expectations about actions that are likely to
come next in the story.

2. *Expectation fails.* The predictions contained in a structure such as
PROVIDE-SERVICE are about the behavior of the participants in a situation governed by that structure. Thus, among other things, we predict
that someone who has voluntarily assumed the SERVER role in that
structure will do what he has been asked to do if he can and if what he
has been asked is within the domain of the area in which he normally
provides his service. In the steak story, making steak rare is within the
range of abilities of the SERVER, yet she has failed to do so. Thus we
have an expectation failure. Our thesis is that such failures must be explained. An understander who does not attempt to explain such failures
will never learn how to cope with any situation that he has not already
coped with. Since we are not born with a complete set of processing
structures, a non-explanation driven system would fail to develop at all
and thus would never understand anything other than whatever was handled by the innate structures it started out with. In other words, without
the ability to explain expectation failures, no memory would be of any
use for very long. Thus, this explanation finding behavior is fundamental
to understanding.

3a. *Assess implicit belief.* The next problem is to explain why the prediction that was made was in error. Why didn't the server do what she was asked?

There are many possible avenues of explanation here. The SERVER could be feeling hostile, recalcitrant or whatever. There is no way to know which of these is the *correct* explanation. An understander is simply concerned with discovering *one* that is feasible. (I don't know why this is true, but people do seem to be happy with an explanation rather than the *best* explanation.) He can then use this explanation to direct future learning.

What we are trying to do here is to understand how Y got reminded of the barber story. There is a correct explanation in the sense that Y got reminded in some particular way and discovering what way is of interest here. In principle, there is more than one possible explanation; as understanders we need only find one that satisfies us. Here we want to assess how Y understood the steak story. That is, we need to determine a path of explanation that could lead a **steak story processor** to his memory of the barber story. Given a multiplicity of possible explanations, an understander need not concern himself with which one is ultimately correct. From the point of view of attempting to establish the algorithm here, we need only show a possible path.

The first task is to assess the implicit belief held by the actor who has failed to behave as expected. On the road towards constructing that belief, we must make an assumption about what the server might have been thinking. Y in this example chose one particular path of explanation. He assumed that the SERVER intended to do what the SERVEE *wanted*.

3b. *Alternative belief.* The Alternative Belief (AB) generated therefore must explain what could have gone wrong. Here again, there are many possible explanations. Y seems to have used: *SERVER must not believe that SERVEE wants what he said he wants, he must want something less extreme that is more in line with the norm for this service.* The issue then is, how do we actually construct such a belief? We will discuss this shortly.

4. *Find memory.* After the Alternative Belief has been constructed we use it as an index in the memory structure PROVIDE-SERVICE at the point where the prediction that a server does what is asked has broken down. At that point in the memory of Y, is the barber story. It has the above Alternative Belief as its explanation as well. This implies that the AB was constructed previously when the barber story was originally understood and created as the index to that memory.

Kinds of explanations

The kinds of failures there are depend entirely on the kinds of predictions there are. Since predictions can be generated from any knowledge structure, any predicted goal, plan, or action can fail. Thus the question of the kinds of failures there are is not the major problem. Most significant is assessing what explanations can be made. Or to put it another way, how are Alternative Beliefs generated? Since we are proposing that memory is organized in part by Alternative Beliefs, this is clearly a key question.

The first question we can ask, in the process of constructing an explanation, is: why didn't the person do what was expected of him or her? There seems an obvious split in the kinds of explanations one can find with respect to this question. People can fail to do what they should have done because they intended to, or the failure can be because of an error of some kind. Thus, there are two kinds of explanation at this level, Motivational Explanations and Error Explanations.

Motivational Explanations (ME'S) are concerned with figuring out why someone would want to do what he did. To construct such explanations we must attempt to find the goals behind the action performed and attempt to relate that goal to the goal that we thought was operating.

Error Explanations (EE'S) are concerned with establishing, given that the actor had exactly the goal we expected him to have – why he couldn't accomplish that goal. To find the reason why a person fails in an attempt at a goal we must assess the kinds of errors he could have made and attempt to establish an Alternative Belief or personal characteristic that would have resulted in such an error being made.

The first problem in constructing an Alternative Belief then is determining whether a motivational or error explanation is what is necessary. In many cases this is determined somewhat arbitrarily. We can just as easily assume that someone made an error as assume that someone really wasn't trying to do what we thought. However, most situations dictate that we seek EE'S before ME'S, since if we can find no error the problem must be with our assessment of the person's goals. Trying to figure out goals is a highly speculative business at best. Thus, there is no decisive way of knowing that you have succeeded at finding the correct ME. If we look for ME'S before EE'S we are likely to find one and thus never consider the possibility that an error occurred. For some actors however, we can assume that their errors were motivational. This would occur with known enemies for example.

To find an EE we must examine the various standard reasons for an error-based failure. Of course, whatever questions we ask about why an error occurred can be asked at every level of failure. Thus, we can ask why someone didn't do what he should, why he didn't plan what he should have, why he didn't have the right goal, and so on. We shall return to this point later.

The first issue we shall discuss is why a person didn't *do* what we expected. When a person fails to do what we expect him to the reasons can be manifold. In the attempt to construct an EE, that is, once we have assumed that there was an error, we can find the following possible starting points: He may not have understood the situation. He may not have had the resources to do his part. He may not have believed that he should do what you thought he should do. He may not have known what to do. He may have been unable to carry out the correct action.

When we attempt to assess the reason for our expectation failure we must look at each of these criteria and establish which is operating at this point. Briefly then we have:

a)   misperception of situation
b)   lack of resources
c)   disbelief
d)   lack of common sense
e)   lack of ability

From these five possibilities, we can now attempt to narrow the field. In the Steak and the Haircut example, we can easily dismiss (b) and (e) by computing the resources and ability necessary and finding them present. There is nothing nonsensical about the actions of the SERVER, so (d) is not a reasonable choice either. It is then our task to discriminate between (a) and (c). We do this almost arbitrarily in this case. It would not be unreasonable to assume that some misperception of what was expected occurred. The only thing *wrong* about this analysis is that it would fail to produce the **Haircut** episode. As that is only one of many possible responses to that story, all we can say here is that Y did not assume a misunderstanding of what was wanted in his analysis.

In order to explain the **Haircut** reminding then, we assume that Y took the path of choosing (c) as his initial explanation. So, the input to the construction of the AB is *disbelief*. From that must be constructed that *the SERVER must not believe that the SERVEE wants what he said he wants; he must want something less extreme.*

Clearly the first part of this was already constructed by the choice of (c) (disbelief). Thus part of the AB is *the SERVER must not believe that the SERVEE wants what he wants.* This results from the combination of the request, the PROVIDE-SERVICE structure, and the non-compliance with the request. To construct the rest of the actual AB requires us to focus on the right feature of what the SERVER actually provided instead. Here the answer is *somethine less extreme*. Clearly then, the problem here is focussing on the extremeness of *not getting your steak rare enough*. Doing this finishes the construction of the AB.

(This last problem, namely focusing on the extremeness is difficult to accomplish. Knowing what is peculiar about a situation allows us to focus our attention in that direction (Schank, 1978) but the process is non-trivial since in some sense, everything is unique.)

Planning failures

In constructing an AB as part of an EE, then, we must attempt to assess the reason for the prediction failure. Where this process starts depends upon where the prediction came from. In the above case, the prediction came from a rather abstract script-like structure that we called PROVIDE-SERVICE, but predictions can come from other structures as well.

The explanation process differs somewhat when we have a planning failure. Consider case D (The Sand Dollars and the Drunk). Notice that case D is superficially similar to case C (The Walking Aunt). Both are failures to plan optimally. From the point of view of an evolutionary system that develops its memory, we can imagine that D might remind one of C early on in its evolution. That is, when there is only one planning failure, one would be reminded of it when a second planning failure is encountered. With a few but varied kinds of planning failures present, *failure to plan optimally* might well be enough to serve as a reminding index. (We discuss this problem of storage and retrieval in an evolving memory in Part IV.)

In a system that contains a large memory, there should be a great many discriminations that separate these two cases and make them quite different from each other. Here again, the problem is to assess the reasons for the prediction failure. We assume a memory organization where those reasons function as indices attached to the memory structure that generated the prediction. In this case, that structure is a plan.

When a plan is perceived by an understander as being different from expected, there can be a number of reasons why it was different. Again we have a distinction between plans that were different because the goal behind them was different (ME'S) and plans that contained errors in their method of achieving the goal we assumed they had (EE'S). For error explanations of planning failures, the questions to be asked are analogous to those asked above for actions.

When a person fails to plan the way we thought he would it may be due to:

a)   having a different goal than we had thought
b)   lack of information and resources
c)   different perception of optimum strategy
d)   lack of common sense
e)   inability

1.   It is possible that the actor did not err in his planning. We may be in error in our assumption of the goal the actor was trying to fulfill. This, of course, leads us to look for an ME.

2.   In order to plan effectively, you need to know a great deal about what possiblities there are and what the situation is. Such a lack of information can yield bad plans. In addition, as with errors about actions, lack of resources can force one into having to select bad plans.

3.   It is not necessarily true that the plan we expect someone to follow is the same one that he will follow even if we have correctly perceived his goal and his information is the same as ours. He may be able to figure out a better plan (one requiring less effort) than the one we expected.

4.   Lack of common sense. If a planner does not do what we expect it may well be that what seems the most reasonable course of action to us may not seem so to him. He may not care to expend effort, for example. Where we believe hard work to be the necessary step in the solution, our planner may not care to work very hard at achieving his goal. He may choose to take an easy way out. Similarly, he may be so foolish as to plan a harder method because he failed to see the optimal and easier way.

5.   Inability. Here again, a planner may simply be incapable of figuring out what to do.

In case D, we have an instance of (d), lack of common sense. The task for the understander is to perceive the girl who is diving for sand dollars as failing to do what was expected at the plan level. To do this we must be tracking her goal of FIND (Sand Dollars). We expect her to employ LOOK and GET in the appropriate place. When she fails to do this we check (a) through (e) above. We know our perception of her goal to be accurate, X has told her the information of where to look, so she has it and she has the ability as is demonstrable by her diving. So the choice is between (c) and (d). X chose (d).

To construct the AB, we need only attempt to explain her lack of common sense. (Note that this explanation need not be grounded in beliefs. *Drunkenness* or *childishness* may suffice as explanations.) Using the possibility that the easiest plan may appear to her to be the best, we construct the AB. *Use the easiest plan despite information to the contrary.* This is used as an index under the goal of FIND (X). At that point, the drunk and the lamppost are also indexed, they being an instance of the same phenomenon exactly.

The value of such indexing seems clear enough. In the case of our own planning, we want to remember plan-failures so that we do not make the same mistake again. In observing others' plans, we may want to help them if their plans do not vitally affect us, or simply not allow bad planners to get the opportunity to partake in plans that do vitally affect us. For the father in case D, after explaining his daughter's failure, his reminding was rather useless. Drawing the analogy between drunks and small children may be amusing, but the learning there is negligible.

Goal failures

One cannot have an error in a goal in the same way that one can pursue the wrong plan, or do an action that was wrong. Explanations are necessary when goals are involved if we have made a prediction error that was caused by our own problems in correctly assessing a situation. In other words, we need to know what we misunderstood about another person's goal. It is easy to misperceive someone else's goal. We can also believe that someone has the wrong goal for his needs. Perhaps more significantly, we can decide that someone's goals conflict with ours, and are *wrong* in the sense that they affect us negatively.

We seek a motivational explanation when we decide that a person knew exactly what they were doing and made no error. That is, we choose ME'S when there are no possible EE'S. Thus ME'S come into play when explanations are necessary to account for people performing actions that we did not expect, due to our misperception of their goals or motivations behind their plans. ME'S are also relevant when we predict poorly because of a conscious assessment of an actor's goals that turns out to be wrong.

The failure to accurately predict someone's behavior then, can often depend on our failure to accurately assess his goals. We can also fail to be adequately prepared for dealing with a goal that another person turns out to have. These are not failures of prediction exactly. We may not even have been aware that this person had the goal that he had. It is even possible that we might not have been aware of the other person's existence. Nevertheless, we can encounter difficulties in our lives that are the result of our not knowing about another's goals. In those cases, as well as in the cases we have talked about above, we need to record our errors and the explanation of those errors for use in future understanding, and to enable us to learn from those experiences.

As an example of the kind of reminding that is relevant here consider an episode taken from Norman & Schank, 1982. Since the names are printed there, we shall keep them here.

The suckering sequences

Norman and Schank went to one of the cafeterias at the University of California at San Diego for lunch. Schank got into the sandwich line, where the server, a young woman, was slicing pieces of meat off of big chunks of roast beef, ham, corned beef, etc. Schank saw the nice looking piece of meat that was exposed on the side of the cut roast beef, and ordered a roast beef sandwich. However, the server had previously sliced some beef off the side, and she took this previously sliced beef for the sandwich. It wasn't nearly as nice as the meat that was still unsliced.

When they sat down at the table in the dining room, Schank turned to Norman and said, "Boy, have I ever been suckered!" He explained what had happened.

Norman sia, "No, you haven't been suckered, because my impression of the word *suckered* is that it implies a serious attempt to defraud."

"You want a real suckering experience?" Normal asked. "On our trip to Spain, we were driving across the country and we came to this tiny little village. We went in to a little store run by someone who looked just like a gypsy lady. We bought some cheese, and great bread, and really nice looking sausage, and some wine. Then we had it all wrapped up and we drove out of the town. We parked in a secluded location, found a hill with some trees, climbed up to the top and sat down looking out over the beautiful countryside. Then we opened the wine and unwrapped the food. Garbage. All there was was garbage, carefully wrapped garbage. Now that was a suckering experience. The gypsy lady suckered us."

The question here is how Norman got reminded of his *suckering* experience. According to our theory, there had to be some explanation that was indexed under a prediction failure that was used by Norman to retrieve the memory. What failure have we got here? The script necessary for understanding Schank's story went without a hitch. No error was made. Indeed, it was not Norman hearing about the events that transpired that reminded Norman of his story. Rather, it was Norman's reaction to Schank's analysis of what had happened to him that reminded Norman of his story. Norman did not believe that Schank's story was an instance of suckering. This disagreement caused the reminding. Now the question is, "How?"

Norman's disagreement was a disagreement about the goals of the server in the cafeteria. He claimed that she did not have the goal of suckering Schank. Schank did not believe that she had that goal either and they later argued about the meaning of the word *sucker*, but that is not the point here. The point is that Norman believes that *suckering* referred only to the intent to defraud and not to the feeling of having been suckered. Because he believed this, he constructed in his head a scenario in which a server served food to a customer that turned out to be different (in a negative way) from what he expected. *Different from what he expected* is, of course, the key item in memory. Such differences must be explained. Norman had constructed an explanation of his gypsy incident that had her goal being poorly assessed as *participate in normal food seller script* where it was actually *use ruse of food seller script to cheat customer out of money*.

In creating a scene in his head that corresponded to his definition of suckering, he created a scenario with an expectation failure that needed explanation. In constructing an ME for that scenario, he came across a memory that had that ME as its index, hence the reminding.

It is important to point out here that Norman's suckering and Schank's story both involve not only misperceived goals and the feeling of being suckered, but the situation of being served food as well. These correspond to an identity of context (food serving as the initial memory organizer for prediction and understanding), prediction failure (resulting in feeling suckered) and explanation (misperceived goals). This latter identity is between Norman's belief in what suckering would have been (that is, not Schank's actual story because he didn't view that as suckering) and Norman's experience with the gypsy.

Summing up

We have outlined here a way of storing and finding memories based on prediction failures. Intrinsic to such a scheme must be a set of structures in memory that generate predictions for use in processing (understanding). The next question is, *What are the structures that memory uses to process inputs and store memories?* Once we have isolated a sensible set of these structures, our next step, considering what we have proposed here, will be to show how such structures are selected for processing, how memories are organized within them, and how failure-driven memories are used for explanation, generalization, and learning. Finally, we shall have to show how reminding can cause these structures to change.

The examples we used here were all situations in which the person being reminded had the possibility of modifying his memory as a result of his reminding experience. Having had an expectation fail, and having had to explain that failure, the individual was then in the position of having to alter his mental structures in some way. The point is simply this: reminding is, in many cases, the impetus to the automatic modification of one's memory structures. Reminding is thus very closely related to understanding and learning. And, most significantly, it is from failures that we learn the most. A memory that gets what it expects every time would never develop in any interesting way. Reminding, expectation failure, and learning, are all intimately connected.

4 Cross-contextual reminding

There are three different kinds of reminding that are relevant for generalization and learning in processing. These different remindings occur at different points during processing with different purposes. They are:

Structure-exemplification

In the initial part of processing, we must find a relevant processing structure. Thus, we must choose a restaurant script or some other high level structure as a source of predictions. Often the selected structure is very tightly linked to a particular episode in memory. It follows that in some cases the best available structure will be that specific episode. One would thus get reminded at that point in processing. This type of reminding occurs, therefore, before any deviation from normal experience, or any expectation failure.

Failure explanation

In Chapter 3 we described reminding that is caused by the need to explain an expectation failure. This kind of reminding occurs when a processing structure has been selected, and an expectation from that structure has failed, and an explanation has been created.

Intentional planning-aids

Sometimes we seek answers to questions we have posed to ourselves, and, in finding those answers we get reminded. The other two types of reminding noted above are remindings that occur unintentionally. We just get reminded in the normal course of doing something else in processing. However, there are times when we are quite deliberately searching memory for something. When we do not know exactly what we were looking for, sometimes we will find an episode that we did not consciously realize we had, yet which turns out to be what we were looking for after all. When what we were doing was attempting to follow a plan, or create our own, we have Intentional Planning-Aids Reminding.

When we create or follow an elaborate plan to achieve some goal, we have implicitly made a prediction that our plan will achieve that goal. Predictions can be made at all levels of the understanding process, but one of the most important kinds of predictions we make is the eventual outcome of a sequence of events. When we observe the plans and actions of others, it is often important to us to be able to assess how things will turn out. When we are doing our own planning, we want to be reminded of those memories to predict what will happen if we use the plan we are considering.

Predicting outcomes

What we are predicting in those structures are outcomes. Because predicting outcomes is of great utility in our lives, it too helps to organize memory. As before, when our predictions fail, we can expect to find memories of prior failures available so that we can make correct future predictions by making appropriate generalizations about the reasons for our prediction failures. Also as before, key questions are: how are failures of this type to be explained, and what kinds of structures are such predictions likely to reside in?

There are actually two kinds of failures worth noting here. As before, what we expect to happen can fail to happen. This is a standard expectation failure. Another failure worth remembering occurs when a set of events result in an outcome that is undesirable, even if anticipated. We may want to note such patterns of events so that we can avert their expected, but undesirable, outcome. Thus, we would expect memories to be organized by such experiences also.

Thus, in processing new inputs, we are not only attempting to understand what happened, but why it happened. An intelligent understander is seeking to learn from his experiences, to draw new conclusions, to make sense of the world. When an expectation failure occurs we ask ourselves why. Similarly, when a disaster occurs, we want to know why. Consider, as an example, President Carter's statements in 1979 about the Russian presence in Afghanistan. He alluded then to the Munich conference of 1938. "No appeasement this time – stop them now" seemed to be the point.

The question for us is: How is an input processed so as to draw out the *appeasement led to disaster* episode from memory? It cannot be simply a question of finding relevant plans and goals. Finding plans and goals means understanding what the Russians are doing. Understanding what the Russians are doing in a deep sense, however, implies recognizing what they might want, what the eventual outcome might be. Carter is saying that understanding the Russians requires understanding the Nazis. How do we grasp that this is his real meaning?

To understand in this sense, we must ask questions about outcomes and steps towards outcomes of events and patterns of events that we hear about or see. By accessing our memories at just the right time and in just the right way, we can view the Russians' actions, and our reactions, in terms of **appeasement at Munich.** How does this happen?

Throughout this book, we have been developing the thesis that inputs are not processed by totally abstract structures such as goals, scripts, and so on. We have argued that such structures are really organizers of epi-sodic memory. Within each abstraction of a script or goal are sets of episodes organized by that structure. In order to get these memories out, we must find the correct index, or cue, under which these memories have been stored.

It seems obvious what the indices are in this example. We have an *aggressive enemy,* an *invasion,* and a setting of *peacetime.* The question is: what kinds of structures in memory are these likely to be useful in search-ing? In addition, how do we find the relevant structures?

To answer these questions, we can consider some alternative situations and see if they would have been likely to remind us of **appeasement in Munich.** For example, suppose the Dutch invaded Luxembourg, citing a centuries-old claim to the land. Would there be cries of *Stop them now or else we'll have another Munich?* The answer seems clearly to be *no.* There is no match possible between Nazi Germany and Holland unless Holland is characterized in a way that is quite out of keeping with how the Dutch are viewed by Americans.

Now consider an instance where a slumlord is buying up decrepit build-ings that he is using as houses of prostitution. In each case, he makes a deal with the authorities that this will be the last one he'll buy if they just leave him alone to conduct his business. Then, later, he says he needs just one more. This circumstance is much closer in spirit to the Munich situa-tion. Further, understanding it would be enhanced if one had access to the moral drawn from **appeasement in Munich.**

It seems reasonable to suppose that the slumlord example might re-mind an interested processor of *Munich* whereas the *Dutch* example would not. In order for the *slumlord* reminding to occur, a very abstract structure must be available. This structure is rooted in the very nature of goal-based processing, namely the need to know why something is happening the way it is. Whenever we note that a goal is operating, we ask, as we said in Schank and Abelson (1977), what the reason or motivation for that goal is. In Schank and Abelson (1977), we postulated that the motivator was a *theme*. If such an answer were sufficient, then processing would end there. We would be happy to say that the Russians satisfied the *aggressor* theme or some such and be done with it.

This is not an adequate answer. As understanders, we seek explanations in terms of our experience. We ask ourselves, "What prior experiences do I have that are like this?" People need to relate what they are currently processing to what they have already processed in order to feel satisfied that they have really understood what was going on. Telling someone the facts of a situation never gives them the picture that a story that embodies those same facts would. This is why Carter encoded his message the way he did. It follows then, that people must have the ability to find experiences in their episodic memories by searching some set of structures that encode those episodes.

Whatever structures are available in memory to help here, it is clear that they must be written in the most general of terms. For the **slumlord** example to remind you of *Munich,* either an organizing structure that contains expectations such as *aggressor wants more* must be available, or one must have the ability to generate such a structure when needed. To put this another way, in order to learn across experiences that have different contexts, noncontextually-based structures must exist in memory. The expectations derived from such a structure must be made in terms with a fairly general scope. That is, it cannot be that a memory structure containing expectations about **slumlords** will somehow happen to contain the *Munich* episode within it.

One problem here then is finding such a structure. We could make the argument that both *Russia* and *slumlord* are somehow pre-categorized as *aggressors*. If this were the case, then *aggressor* could be a thematic structure that functioned in the same way that we have suggested that goals and scripts function, as organizers of actual episodes.

When is **slumlord** categorized as an aggressor? The answer is, after he has done the aggression – and thus after the reminding experience of *Munich* has already come to light. That is, it was the reminding that classified the slumlord as an aggressor. *The input itself contributed to the categorization.*

The real commonality here is the resultant prediction. That is, in each case we expect a certain outcome, and these outcomes are the same. We expect that the actor who only wants a little now, will want more in the future. In processing both the *Russia* case and the **slumlord** case, we are considering the goals of the actors. As we speculate about future goals, we ask the question "When will it stop, why won't they want more?" This question expresses an expectation about future actions that is contained in the abstract structure that has been activated at that point. This question serves as an index within that structure that causes the *Munich* experience to come to mind. We do not ask this question in the *Dutch* case because a different structure is active in processing that story. Thus, no reminding occurs.

We are saying that reminding across contexts can depend on speculations about possible outcomes. Whereas before, the index to memory that found relevant memories was an explanation of odd behavior, here the index is a question or speculation about future actions. In failure-driven reminding, we sought explanations because an incorrect expectation had been generated by an operating knowledge structure. We sought an explanation for our error. Here there is no error, merely an inquiry to know more. Thus we must concern ourselves with the following issues:

1. Why do we worry about predicting outcomes?
2. What structure in memory is directing processing at the point where the predictions are made?

The answer to the first question depends upon our conception of the nature of the understanding process. We have claimed that expectations are the key to understanding. In a great many instances, these expectations are sitting in a particular spot in memory, awaiting the call to action. Frequently they are prepackaged like scripts. That is, the expectations have been made before and are waiting around to be made again.

Often, however, generating relevant expectations is not so simple. Sometimes we are on relatively new ground. That is, on the basis of prior experience, it is not always all that obvious what to expect. Now, there are two possibilities here. In such situations we can simply not expect anything. We can just take what comes. Alternatively, we can work hard at creating expectations by whatever means we may have available.

The former possibility is quite feasible. It is quite reasonable to suppose that some people do go through situations having no idea what to expect and just taking it as it comes. While it is certainly possible to expect nothing, it seems likely that there is great value to generating expectations in novel situations because it facilitates learning from those situations. Learning means altering existing structures. *If we have no expectations, we cannot easily notice that our prior view of the world was in error and needed to be corrected. That is, we will not alter any memory structures as a result of a given experience.*

What we want to do, then, is attempt to figure out what will happen in any situation we encounter. To put this another way, when we hear that someone has a goal, we must attempt to figure out why they have that goal, what goal they might have next, what pattern their behavior implies and so on. In a sense then, we are plotting possible scenarios in our heads about everything we see. We are attempting to imagine what will happen next. To do so, we must construct a model of how things will turn out. (This model can often be quite wrong, of course.) Sometimes, during the construction of this model, we come across memories that embody exactly the state of affairs that we were constructing. When we reach those experiences we have an instance of Outcome-Driven Reminding.

So, the answer to the first question above is that such an inquiry is made whenever the events that are taking place are perceived to have a possible effect on the understander (or a person the understander cares about or identifies with). That is, when we hear about goal-directed behavior, we will attempt to predict an outcome of that behavior if it can possibly affect us. To do this, we must have asked ourselves about the goals that were being pursued, found the plans that seemed to be operating, and used them to assess the likely outcome of those plans.

The real problem here is how to generate a question such as *When will their demands stop?* and how to use that question to find a relevant memory. For our knowledge of goals, plans and outcomes to be accessible at the right times, that knowledge must be stored in a processing structure. Thus, a processing structure must be capable of providing us with possible outcomes for the set of situations organized by that structure. In order to find a relevant memory in a processing structure, we must select an appropriate structure first. The question that we formulate about outcomes then, must enable us to find a relevant memory that is organized in terms of a processing structure that is already active. It would be of little use if we queried memory for relevant experiences on which to create expectations if those experiences were stored in structures different from those we were looking in at the time. The kinds of structures we imagine are ones that organize outcomes in terms of goals.

To see what structure we could possibly have here, we need to examine what information it is that we know at this point. First, we know that an actor has taken something that he wanted. Second, and most important, we have assessed that actor as having evil intentions with respect to what he wants to do with what he now possesses. When these two features are identified, we claim that a high level structure has been found under which memories are organized. (We call this structure a Thematic Organization Packet or TOP. TOPS will be explained in Chapter 7. Here we will simply note some of this particular TOP'S properties.)

We shall call the TOP-level structure that is active here, **Possession Goal; Evil Intent** or PG;E1 for short. The first problem we have in using any knowledge structure is selecting it. In this case, all we have had to have been doing is noting goals and speculating on the reasons for those goals. In the slumlord story we are told those reasons. For Russia, we would need to have Russia precategorized as an actor with evil intents.

Once such a structure has been found, we expect that it will function much like any high level knowledge structure. That is, it will be a source of predictions about what we can expect will happen within the context of that structure. What expectations are we likely to find organized by this TOP?

Any TOP is a collection of information about what usually happens within a certain high-level context. In general, three kinds of information are stored within a given TOP. First, we have *expectational information*. TOPs provide a set of expectations about what may happen next under various circumstances within that TOP. Second, we have *static information*. This is knowledge of the state of the world that describes what is happening when that TOP is active. Thus, for example, we know about the feelings and attitudes of the participants in the TOP. Third, we have *relational information*. This includes characterizations of the world that help us link a TOP to other structures in memory. For example, the word *bully* naturally comes to mind in the TOP being discussed. This characterization of an actor as a bully may serve to link information similarly characterized but stored in different TOPs. Most of all, of course, a TOP is a set of memories organized by the TOP.

TOPs are searched in order to create a variety of expectations, including predictions about the outcome of the event being processed. We make a prediction about outcomes by supplying the relevant TOP with some index that gets us to notice a relevant memory organized by that TOP. That memory gives us something with which we can make a prediction about an outcome. Here there is no failure of any kind in the processing of the input. What failure there might be is present in the memory that one is reminded of; that is, our failure to plan adequately last time (in the Munich experience). Thus, the problem here is not one of error-correction. Rather, an understander must use his knowledge of past experience to help him through a situation. In other words, he needs to assess a probable outcome because he is being called upon to make a decision of some type. Getting reminded of a relevant experience will help recall that process. Thus, outcome-driven reminding can be an active part of planning.

Outcomes and reminding

To see the kind of reminding I have in mind here, consider the following four cases. Note that these cases have in common that they are cross-contextual. That is, their similarities are best expressed by common themes or patterns of goals, rather than by similar locations or scripts. It is these kinds of remindings that are most relevant to the prediction of an outcome, and hence to planning.

E. *Romeo and Juliet*

When watching the play *West Side Story* it is quite common for people to be reminded of *Romeo and Juliet*.

F. *Munich and Afghanistan*

(This is what we have been discussing.)

G. *Nixon and the Mayor of New Haven*

In New Haven politics there are sometimes strained town-gown relations. The past mayor was *Yale-affiliated*. The current mayor ran on a more *anti-Yale* platform but after his election he established better relations with Yale than his predecessor had. This reminded X of President Nixon's anti-communism stance and his ability to make friends with both Russia and China.

H. *Back Street*

The movie *Back Street* describes an affair that began when old lovers who had intended to marry, but couldn't due to a mishap, met after many years. When the mishap occurred, X was *not* reminded of *Romeo and Juliet*. When the lovers discussed the accidental situation, X found himself saying *well he should have informed her of his plans*. This reminded X of *Romeo and Juliet*.

These four cases have in common the failure of a predicted outcome.

In E, we predict that Romeo and Juliet will live happily ever after due to her clever plan to take false poison.

In F, we predict that giving in to the Nazis will let them get what they want and stop bothering us.

In G, we predict that a politician running on a platform of anti-Y, goes after Y upon election.

In H, we note that the hero predicted that his friend would arrive and they would get married, but she never arrived.

The above cases provide a view of processing that has an understander continually searching for *how it will all turn out in the end*. It is not sufficient to just say that we are attempting to predict outcomes. We must look at how we could predict an outcome.

The first problem again, is establishing what high level knowledge structure is being employed.

Let us consider case E, the problem of *West Side Story* reminding a viewer of *Romeo and Juliet*. Adopting the point of view that:

1. We are constantly searching for outcomes
2. Outcomes are to be found by an index in a TOP

then in order for *West Side Story* to remind someone of *Romeo and Juliet* he must have been using a memory structure which contained the *Romeo and Juliet* memory while understanding the story.

Thus we can ask:

1. What patterns are around to be noticed?
2. What TOP is used?
3. What indices are used in that TOP to find the outcome?

Here again, a good way to approach these questions is to see what else might remind you of Romeo and Juliet. There seem to be a number of key factors that might contribute to a *Romeo and Juliet reminding*. These are:

1. young lovers
2. objections of parents
3. an attempt to get together surreptitiously
4. a false report of death
5. the false report causes a real death of one of the lovers

Now, one thing to do here is to attempt to change some of these factors to test our intuitions about whether the reminding would occur. For example, suppose the lovers were of the same sex. This might be considered a *gay Romeo and Juliet* so sex is probably not a relevant index to the TOP, nor a relevant part of the TOP. Suppose the lovers were old and it was their children who objected. Or suppose, for young lovers, their respective ethnic groups objected. It seems reasonable to suppose that we would still get the *Romeo and Juliet* reminding. (In fact, one of those is *West Side Story.)*

Suppose we didn't have lovers, but say had business partners. Even there, if the rest of the story followed, *Romeo and Juliet* might come to mind.

Suppose there was no attempt to get together; then there is no story clearly, so that is crucial. Similarly, suppose there was no false report of death. This seems critical, but, for the business partners, suppose this were transformed into a false report of a merger or bankruptcy. In that case, the *Romeo and Juliet* plot might still be there. The impossibility of righting things afterwards seems rather important, though. The death, although it probably could be changed to some figurative death (like bankruptcy) seems critical.

So what are we left with? We have two people trying to get together, being thwarted by outside opposition, eventually resulting in a false report of a tragedy that results in an actual tragedy for the other.

Let's call the TOP here **mutual goal pursuit against outside opposition.** Two indices are *false report* of tragedy and *tragedy resulting from false report.* Either of these indices can be used to find the *Romeo and Juliet* memory. Thus, the outcome could be predicted by *false report.* Another index is the outcome, so it can also serve to produce the reminding experience.

Now, we will attempt to merge all this with the notions we discussed in the last chapter. Roughly, the algorithm presented for Failure-Driven reminding was:

> Process according to knowledge structures
> Detect prediction failures
> Explain failure
> Create alternative account
> Access memory through belief

In the cases we have been discussing, the TOPs selected were PG;EI, and Mutual Goal Pursuit Against Outside Opposition (MG;OO). Comparing this to the failure-driven cases discussed in Chapter 3, we can see that the indices must be different. In those cases explanations were created to account for expectation failures. Those explanations were the indices to memory. Here, as we shall see, the indexing mechanism works differently.

Once a TOP has been selected for processing, we begin to generate expectations. Expectations are generated by using appropriate indices to find specific episodes organized by that TOP. The indices are selected through a variety of techniques (described in Chapter 10) by examining various features of the input story, or by asking oneself general questions about the TOP, the answers to which can serve as indices. The trick in generating this latter type of index is to ask questions that have answers that have already been used as indices. One method for doing this is to attempt to solve the *problem* of the TOP. Since TOPs are collections of goal combinatins in various circumstances, they have, associated with them, a problem. In PG;EI it is how to react to the evil actor. In MG;OO it is achieving the mutual goal. Imagining a particular solution can bring to mind specific episodes that tried that solution in the past.

In case E, once MG;OO has been selected as the relevant TOP, any number of indices that describe specific, unusual features of *West Side Story,* will help to pull out the *Romeo and Juliet* episode from memory. One of these indices, for example, is *false report of death of the co-planner.* This gives us the actual memory, i.e., the path to *Romeo and Juliet* is provided by that index. Thus the prediction here is that any story employing the above TOP and the above index will remind you of *Romeo and Juliet.* The advantage of being reminded of *Romeo and Juliet* here is that one can speculate, on the basis of that past episode, how the current episode being processed will turn out. In watching plays this is of little import, but in real life situations knowing how a similar set of circumstances turned out can be extremely significant.

Now let's consider case F (Munich and Afghanistan). The TOP is PG;EI as we indicated earlier. In this case we are attempting to formulate a reasonable response to the PG;EI. PG;EI is, by its nature, a TOP that we must respond to. Expectations within PG;EI thus involve possible responses and the outcomes of those responses. For *Romeo and Juliet,* we need do nothing other than observe, but in this case Carter wanted to take action and have the American people approve. The understanding tasks are different here. In essence, we are trying to remind ourselves of the most relevant memory we have to help us react to this situation. To do this, we must create indices that will lead us to the potential solution paths. In this way we can mentally try the solution and see what memories we are reminded of that employed that solution. In other words, in cases where we must compose a response to someone else's action that can be characterized by a TOP, we postulate *conditional outcomes* that we mentally *try out* as possible responses.

In case F, one possible plan, and therefore one possible index to PG;EI, is the null plan: *Provide no opposition.* Using this as an index in PG;EI will help retrieve the memory of the Nazis and Munich. That is, it is as if the question were posed to memory, "When an aggressor has asked for more territory and no opposition was provided, what has happened?"

Memory answers the question by providing a prior episode whose outcome was a series of escalating demands. From this memory we can then predict future failures if *provide no opposition* is the course chosen.

The moral here is that if you want to influence people's thinking indirectly, give them a situation that can be characterized by a TOP, and a possible index to that TOP. People will use that index to find a memory. If that memory has negative consequences, they will then begin to believe that a course of action other than the one expressed by the index should be taken. In a sense then, the point of getting us to think about *provide no opposition* as a possible plan is to cause us to counterplan. *Provide no opposition* fails, so something else must work.

After an index has yielded a bad effect, if the problem we are processing is our own, we try to create an alternative plan. To do so, we must identify the causes of the failure of the original episode. Clearly for *Romeo and Juliet* this is of little use for us to do as understanders. Yet, many people find themselves incapable of not doing it. We tend to try to create an alternative plan by negating one or more of the conditions in the failed plan. In F, the obvious thing to do is to negate *provide no opposition* by making it *provide opposition*. This new plan is equivalent to an explanation for the failure of the prior plan. Thus, for this kind of reminding, explanations are the last item produced since they are post hoc.

Now let us consider case G. This reminding came about because X was being asked to evaluate the performance of the mayor of New Haven. X was forced, in attempting to analyze the mayor's performance, to rely on previous information. In other words, X tried to find an episode in memory that would provide a valid analogy.

In G then, it appears that X was asking himself to evaluate the behavior of the mayor. The TOP *achieve success, utilize power* is active. That TOP predicts that the mayor will plan to do what he has said he would do. **Hurt Enemies** is one thing that is expected. It is thus a plan, that, in conjunction with the index of *political power through elective office* brings the memory of Nixon to mind. But Nixon did not hurt his ideological enemies in the international sphere; he only bothered with his personal political enemies. This information is then used to note the similarity with the mayor of New Haven and to start the process of post-hoc explanation. In other words, upon evaluation of these two inputs, a new memory structure might be created that provided expectations about certain types of candidates for office.

The most important thing we must do in Outcome-Driven Reminding is create a new belief or conclusion that will better enable future understanding. Here, we must be able to create a belief like *Those who get elected attacking Y are good people to make friends with Y*. It is this conclusion that is most obviously drawn from the two instances and it is this kind of creative generalization that we seek to make. The creation of new structures from old ones that have failed is an important part of learning.

Finally, let's consider case H. The movie *Back Street* has little in common with *Romeo and Juliet*. When X saw that movie he was not reminded of *Romeo and Juliet,* at least not initially. The basis of the plot of *Back Street* is a marriage plan. The hero does not inform the heroine of the plan. They fail to meet at the appointed time. Subsequently, they each marry someone else, and then end up having an affair when they meet later in life. When X thought about their initial failure to meet, well after the actual scene, he found himself saying to himself "Well, he should have made sure that his plan was known to his lover, and then it would have worked out." It was this explanation of what had gone wrong that reminded X that that was the conclusion he had come to about what went wrong for Juliet. That is, both stories lead one to the same conclusion about planning in a MG;OO.

To understand *Back Street,* it is necessary, at one level of understanding, to figure out why what went wrong in a person's life ·went wrong. Clearly, it is not absolutely necessary to do this in order to understand; it is necessary if one wants to understand well, however.

In the course of understanding *West Side Story,* we had to get reminded of *Romeo and Juliet,* so to speak. In following the course of events in the story, we get reminded as we access a TOP and attempt to predict an outcome. In case H, we do not even realize that a MG;OO is present because it is not obvious to the viewer of the movie what the hero's plan is. Later, when we realize that things have gone awry, we could decide to think about why if we want to, but that is not necessary. When we attempt to understand what we are hearing or seeing at a deeper level, that is, when we decide to ask ourselves why some event occurred, we then must access the relevant TOP, find the plan that was used, and note the outcome. When we seek to explain the outcome, we come upon related memories, as before, that have been indexed in various ways. Here we see that one possible index is the conclusion that we draw from the experience. That is, X realized that the hero should have been sure his coplanner was informed in a MG;OO, and that being the conclusion he came to for *Romeo and Juliet,* he was reminded of that story. Thus, conclusions can also be indices.

Drawing conclusions

To predict outcomes we must be able to draw conclusions from what has happened. One way to do this is to take two memories that we have found to be in common by reminding and to create from them a new rule that can be used in the understanding process. We want to learn from prior failures. We attempt to predict an outcome, and, coming upon a related prior memory, draw a conclusion that causes us to modify our behavior in order to avert the same problem we encountered last time.

In general then, what we want to do is make a generalization from any reminding example that will help us next time around. Consider then, the generalizations that might be drawn from the examples cited above:

F.   When dealing with an aggressor who wants more, draw the line quickly.
G.   If you want peace with X, support politicians who are anti-X.
H.   Be sure that your coplanner is informed of your plans.

In each of these examples then, what we want to do is derive a rule that can be placed at an appropriate point in memory to aid us next time. To do this we must isolate the reason for the outcome related failure and index in terms of that reason.

Simply stated then, we are proposing that in Outcome-Driven Reminding the task is to find a memory that will help in planning a reaction to a current problem. This kind of reminding is much more intentional than Failure-Driven Reminding. Here, we are not only trying to understand why someone did what they did, we are also trying to modify plans for achieving goals. Thus, while FDM is driven by expectations involving actions, ODM is driven by expectations involving plans and goals. The consequences for a system that learns from such remindings are thus more profound in ODM since such remindings can effect generalizations that cause us to avoid possible dangers caused by bad planning.

Reminding is the key to our understanding. When we find a memory during the course of processing, the act of finding that memory forces us to modify our existing knowledge structures. This modification takes the form of changing the expectations in the structures, or of creating new structures. Since structures and their expectations are forms of generalization in memory, this alteration process is a component part of an overall process of generalization.

In the remainder of this book, therefore, we have three significant issues to address:

1. What structures are there in memory?
2. How are these structures altered to modify expectations and create new generalizations?
3. How can we find the right structures and memories held in those structures so as to begin the process of expectation and reminding?

We will attempt to answer these questions in what follows. The conclusion so far is this: Reminding is a ubiquitous phenomenon in memory. Often, a reminding is illustrative of previous processing in memory that has attempted to record failures of various kinds together with the explanation of those failures. Such failures come from expectations that we make about the way things are likely to happen, and from our desires about the way we want events to turn out. These expectations are created at all levels of processing. People are constantly trying to figure out what will happen and what to do about it. They look for patterns and attempt to solidify those patterns by creating structures in their memories that encode various sets of expectations.

Any theory of memory therefore must concentrate on the nature of the memory structures that encode expectations. We consider that issue next.

Part II

Structures in memory

5   The kinds of structures in memory

The nature of understanding

Two people can have the same experience, yet encode it differently. They can each see the same thing as confirmation of quite different beliefs. In a sense, we see things we are prepared to see. Or, in other words, we see things in terms of what we have already experienced. The structures that one has available in memory are the embodiment of one's experiences. We understand in terms of the structures that we have available. And, the structures we have available reflect how we have understood things in the past. Thus, it is critical to carefully reflect upon the nature of memory structures.

In Chapter 2, we discussed how a Burger King trip might *remind* someone of McDonald's. What kind of reminding is this? There is no obvious failure here. Basically, there are two possibilities. If McDonald's is encoded in memory as a failure of our normal expectations about restaurants, Burger King would constitute a similar failure, and reminding would occur. On the other hand, McDonald's could be encoded in memory as an entity in its own right, apart from knowledge about restaurants in general. In that case the natural processing of Burger King should lead to the same structure that encoded McDonald's. Use of a structure that has a unique referent (McDonald's) will cause one to be reminded of that referent.

Understanding an input means finding the closest approximation in one's past experience to the input and coding it in terms of the previous memory with an index that indicates the difference between the new input and the old memory. Understanding, then, implies using expectation failures driven by prototypical memories or specific memories indexed under prototypical memories. Understanding is reminding (or re-cognizing, to take that word literally) and reminding is finding the correct memory structure to process an input. Our major problem then, in formulating a theory of understanding, is to find out what the requisite high level memory structures might look like.

How do high level structures get built?

To answer this question let us digress for a moment to the topic of how scripts or similar structures might come to exist in the human mind.

Children, as we have noted in Schank and Abelson (1977) and as Nelson and Gruendel (1979) note, learn scripts from a very early age. We hypothesize that the basic entity of human understanding is what we have termed the *personal script.* Personal scripts are our private expectations about how things proceed in our own lives on a day to day or minute to minute basis. In the beginning, a child's world is organized solely in terms of personal scripts, i.e., his private expectations about getting his diaper changed or being fed or going shopping. Such expectations abound for children and children can be quite vocal when these expectations are violated. The child who has gotten a piece of candy at every grocery store visit will complain wildly when he does not get it at the current grocery store. These expectations are not limited to such positively anticipated experiences however. Trifles such as taking a different route to the same place or not being placed in the same seat as last time are very important to children and serve as reminders to us of the significance of personal scripts in children's lives.

As time goes on children begin to notice that other human beings share some, but not all, of their expectations. When a child discovers, for example, that his personal restaurant script is also shared by other people, he can resort to a new method of storage for restaurant information. He can rely on a standardized restaurant script with certain personal markings that store his own idiosyncratic points of view. That is, he can begin to organize his experiences in terms that separate what is peculiar to his experience from what is shared by his culture.

For example, adults know that getting in a car is not part of the restaurant script. However, this may be a very salient feature of a child's personal restaurant script. It is very important for a child to learn that the car experience must be separated from the restaurant experience so that he can recognize a restaurant without having gone there by car and so that he can understand and talk about other people's restaurant experiences. Thus, the child must learn to reorganize his memory store according to cultural norms.

Adults do not abandon personal scripts as important organizational entities. We still expect the doorman to say good morning as he opens the door or expect the children to demand to be played with immediately after dinner or whatever sequences we are used to. We may no longer cry when these things do not happen, but we expect them nonetheless. These expectations pervade our lives just as they did when we were children.

We continue to reorganize information that we have stored indefinitely. New experiences are constantly being reorganized on the basis of similar experiences and cultural norms. The abstraction and generalization process for knowledge acquired through experience is thus a fundamental part of adult understanding. When you go to the dentist for the first time, everything in that experience is stored either as a single, isolated chunk, or in terms of experiences (with doctors perhaps) that seem similar. Repeated experiences with the same dentist or other dentists, and descriptions of others' experiences with dentists serve to reorganize the original information in terms of what is peculiar to your dentist, dentists in general, yourself in dental offices, and so on. The reorganization process never stops. When similarities between doctors and dentists are seen, a further reorganization can be made in terms of health care professionals. When doctors' and lawyers' similarities are extracted, yet another memory organization point emerges. The key to understanding is this continual creation of new high level structures where the essential similarities between different experiences are recorded.

In this view, one's concept of an event is simply the collocation of one's repeated encounters with that event. After only one trip to the dentist, the dentist who treated you is your prototypical dentist. Over time, your concept of a dentist evolves. Similar or identical parts of the various dentist experiences you have had are abstracted into structures representing the generalized prototype. New experiences are then stored in terms of their differences from the prototype.

To begin our look at the kinds of high level structures that there must be let us consider a possible story about a trip to the dentist.

The first question we wish to address with this example is what knowledge is used in processing the various parts of the story. The second question is what memory looks like after this story has been processed. Since memory structures and processing structures are the same thing, it should be clear that any story has the potential for altering memory, especially if it differs from the prototypes that are being used to process it. In particular, any failures of expectations arising from those prototypes will in some way cause an alteration to memory.

Previously (Schank & Abelson, 1977), we have said that the structure that would handle a visit to the dentist was the DENTIST script. The DENTIST script would contain a list of events normally found in visits to the dentist, connected together causally. In addition, we allowed *tracks* of such a script to represent the alternative sequences of events that could take place. Under this conception of a script, the script's primary role was as an orderer of scenes, each of which in turn served to order events within those scenes. Each action encoded in a script thus served as an expectation that memory was making about incoming input.

What of all this do we wish to keep in our present conception of things, and what do we believe to be missing? The first change that we have been suggesting transforms the notion of a script from a passive data structure from which expectations are hung, to an active memory structure that changes in response to new input. The failure of expectations derived from a script will cause indices to be placed in the script at the failure point. When similar failures are noted, the memory indexed by them directs processing at that point. We have already discussed this to some extent previously and will have more to say about this self-organization process in Chapter 8. The key point here is that scripts are active memory structures.

What else is missing from our prior conception of scripts? As we discussed in Chapter 1, there is a serious problem that was demonstrated by the Bower, Black and Turner (1979) experiments, namely the problem of determining the right level of information to be stored in scripts. It seems reasonable to suppose that what we know about dentist's waiting rooms is just what we know about waiting rooms in general, and is not specific to dentists. A waiting room in a dentist's office is likely to be more or less identical to that of a doctor's office. An event that occurs within the setting of a waiting room is more likely to be remembered as an event that occurred in a waiting room than one that occurred in a dentist's office. Similarly then, we can expect that what we know about waiting rooms may apply in a great many other circumstances: lawyers' offices, for instance.

The same thing is true of many of the other activities involved in a visit to a dentist. *Paying the bill* or *getting to the dentist's office* involves knowledge sources and hence memories that may not involve dentists at all. We use what we know about these two things to help us understand a visit to the dentist, but there is no reason to assume that the memories and memory structures that we use in these situations are stored in any way that connects them intimately to what we know about dentists. To drive to a dentist's office we do not need to know anything about dentists except how to get to that particular dentist's office.

What we are proposing, then, is that a lot of that knowledge that we would previously have stored as part of the dentist script is, in reality, part of other memory structures that get used in understanding a story involving a dentist visit. Such a proposal has two obvious ramifications. First, this view implies that scripts do not exist in the form we had previously proposed. While it may be possible to collect all the expectations we have about a complex event into one complex structure that contains everything we know about visits to the dentist, such a structure does not actually exist in memory. Instead, the expectations are distributed in smaller, sharable units. Second, if a diverse set of memory structures are used for processing a story about a visit to a dentist, and if memory structures are the same as processing structures, then it follows that a story about a visit to the dentist will get broken up by memory into several distinct pieces. That is, whatever happens in driving to the dentist's office, if it is of interest to memory, it will be stored as a modification of what we know about driving, not dentists. Each event will be processed by, and stored in terms of, the structure that relates most closely to that event.

Such a scheme has the negative effect of forcing us to use a reconstructive memory to help us recall events that have happened to us. (And, of course, we may not be able to reconstruct everything.) But this negative effect is more than outweighed by the powerful advantage of enabling us to learn by generalizing from experiences by noticing their commonalities. We shall discuss this trade-off more carefully in the remainder of this book.

A third important implication is that there must be some memory structures available whose job it is to connect other memory structures together. In order to reconstruct what has happened to us, and in order to have the relevant structures available for processing when they are needed, memory structures must exist that tie other structures together in the proper order. Even though we have learned to disassociate memories about WAITING ROOM from those specific to DENTIST, we still need to know that dentist visits involve waiting rooms.

Information about how memory structures are ordinarily linked in frequently occurring combinations, is held in a *memory organization packet* or what we shall henceforth call a MOP.

In order to account for reconstructive memory, and the ability to generalize and learn from past experience, I am proposing that a memory structure exists that I call a MOP. It follows from what I have said so far that a MOP is also a processing structure. As a memory structure, the role of a MOP is to provide a place to store new inputs. As a processing structure, the role of a MOP is to provide expectations that enable the prediction of future inputs or inference of implicit events on the basis of previously encountered, structurally similar, events. A MOP processes new inputs by taking the aspects of those inputs that relate to that MOP and interpreting those aspects in terms of the past experiences most closely related to them. Many different high-level memory structures can be relevant at any given time in processing an input, i.e., any of a number of different MOPs may be applicable at one time.

We said in Chapter 1 that scenes hold memories. Scenes are general structures that describe how and where a particular set of actions take place. WAITING ROOM or AIRPORT RENT-A-CAR COUNTER are possible scenes. Scripts (in our new formulation of them) embody specific predictions connected to the more general scene that dominates them. Thus, an individual might have a *$DOCTOR JONES' WAITING ROOM* script that differs in some way from the more general WAITING ROOM scene. Scenes, therefore, can point to scripts that embody specific aspects of those scenes. Scripts can also hold memories that are organized around expectation failures within that script. In this view of scripts, a script is bounded by the scene that contains it. Thus scripts do not cross scene boundaries.

MOPs differ from scenes and scripts in the amount of knowledge they cover and the generality of that knowledge. A script must be limited to a sequence of actions that take place in one physical setting. Similarly, a scene is setting-bounded. But a MOP can contain information that covers many settings. Furthermore, a MOP has a purpose that is not readily inferable from each of the scenes or scripts that it contains. Because of this, memory confusions can take place when it is forgotten which MOP a particular scene-based memory was connected to. This is like remembering what you did without remembering exactly why you were doing it. Some examples of this include remembering an incident that took place while you were driving and being unable to recall where you were driving to, or remembering a waiting room without being able to recall exactly why you were there.

Now it is important to consider how MOPs function in the understanding process. Let us consider the imformation relevant to a visit to a doctor's office. The primary job of a MOP in processing new inputs is to provide relevant memory structures that will in turn provide expectations necessary to understand what is being received. Thus MOPs are responsible for filling in implicit information about what events must have happened but were unstated. At least two MOPs are relevant to processing, memory, and understanding of what a visit to a doctor's office entails. They are: M-PROFESSIONAL OFFICE VISIT and M-CONTRACT.

Each of these MOPs organizes scenes and scripts relevant to the processing of any story involving a visit to a doctor. WAITING ROOM, for example, is one of the scenes in M-PROFESSIONAL OFFICE VISIT (hence-forth M-POV).

The primary function of M-POV is to provide the correct sequencing of the scenes that provide the appropriate expectations for use in processing. In order to create the proper set of expectations, we must recognize what MOPs are applicable. How do we do this? Consider the following story:

I went to the doctor's yesterday. While I was reading a magazine I noticed that a patient who arrived after me was being taken ahead of me. The doctor will probably still overcharge me!

Previously, in our script-based theory we would have said that the first line of this story called in a comprehensive doctor script. We are currently postulating that no such entity should exist in memory as a prestored chunk. A memory that used a high level structure such as *doctor visit* would not be able to take advantage of similarities across experiences. A system that used such structures could never apply what it found in one context to help in another. Thus it would not learn in any truly interesting way. We must be able to remember an experience by retrieving the memories of the pieces that comprised that experience. The alternative (memory storage that contains entire experiences as a distinct unit) would preclude learning across contexts.

In processing the first sentence of this story, what we must do is call in the relevant MOPs insofar as we can determine them, and begin to set up expectations to help in processing the rest of the story. This is done as follows: The phrase *went to the doctor* refers to "doctor", which is something about which we have information. Doctor is a token in memory. For every token in memory, there exists information attached to that token that tells us where to look for further information. Attached to the doctor token is, among other things, information about the MOPs that a doctor, in his role as doctor, is likely to participate in.

The information attached to the doctor token that is relevant to this example is a combination of MOPs and information about the conditions in the world that tell us when those MOPs are likely to be active. This information includes parsing information about what words or concepts in the context **doctor** may help to tell us what MOP may be active. In this case, *PTRANS to doctor* (PTRANS is a primitive action underlying "go" and other verbs; see Schank, 1975) activated the MOP that refers to going to a doctor's office for his professional services. Thus, this activates M-POV. (Saying "John is a doctor" would not activate that M-POV. The activation process is actually more complex than this, but this will suffice for our purposes here.)

M-POV has information attached to it concerning what other MOPs might also be active when M-POV is active. In addition to what we know about visits to a professional's office, we also know quite a bit about why the actors in the various scenes of that MOP do what they do. Knowing this allows us to predict further actions not explicitly part of M-POV. It is in no sense a requisite part of M-POV, for example, that people pay for the service they get. Services can, of course, be free (as doctors' are in various countries). Included as part of M-POV then, is information that, in this person's experience, the MOP M-CONTRACT is activated when M-POV is activated. That is, we know that an implicit contract has been made by patient and doctor and that a bill will be sent as a result of this contract, that the patient will be sued if he doesn't pay and so on. All of this information is part of M-CONTRACT, not M-POV. Thus a MOP carries with it at least two kinds of information: an ordered set of scenes (or placeholders for scenes) and other MOPs that frequently co-occur with it.

A MOP serves to organize a set of scenes and scripts commonly associated with a goal in memory. Thus M-POV organizes what we know about what ordinarily takes place in a visit to a professional's office. It would not have in it anything specific to the higher level goals involved in such a visit. That is, we know that people go to doctors to pursue health-related goals. But that information is not contained in M-POV. Rather, M-HEALTH PROTECTION is also activated by "PTRANS to doctor." As we shall see later on MOPs tend to come in threes. The three active in a doctor visit then are M-HEALTH PROTECTION, M-CON-TRACT, and M-POV. These correspond to personal, societal, and physical MOPs respectively. This three-part division is quite significant and will be explored further in subsequent chapters.

A scene defines a setting, an instrumental goal, and actions that take place in that setting in service of that goal. These actions are defined in terms of specific and generalized memories relating to that setting and goal. For example, *ordering in a restaurant* or *getting your baggage in an airport* are scenes. As long as there is an identifiable physical setting and a goal being pursued with that setting, we have a scene. Two kinds of information are present in a scene. First, we have physical information about what the scene looks like. Information about what was in one's line of sight can be part of one's remembrance of a scene. Second, we have information about the activities that go on in a scene. (We shall look at scenes in more detail in Chapters 6 and 9.)

A script, in our new, narrower, sense, is a sequence of actions that take place within a scene. Many scripts can encode the various possibilities for the realization of a scene. That is, a script instantiates or *colors* a scene.

Scenes contain general information; scripts provide the specifics. This will be explained more carefully in Chapter 6.

Let us look in detail at the structure of two of the MOPs, M-POV and M-CONTRACT.

M-POV has the following structure:

> [get there] + WAITING ROOM + GET SERVICE + PAY
> + [get back]

M-CONTRACT consists of:

> [get contact] + NEGOTIATE + AGREE + DELIVER + PAY

The entities between the plus signs are the structures organized by the MOP. The MOP exists to provide an ordering for these structures. The following structures are organized by MOPs:

Structures organized by MOPs	Denoted	Example
SCRIPTS	$XXX	$HERTZ-COUNTER
SCENES	XXX	RENT-A-CAR COUNTER
PLACE HOLDERS	[xxx]	[get transportation]

Scenes in parentheses are optional and need not occur in every instantiation of that MOP.

Place-holders indicates pieces of the episode for which expectations will be provided by some other knowledge structures. For example, M-POV contains the place-holder [get there]. What we mean here is that a great many MOPs, scenes, or scripts can fit in that spot. If you took a bus to the doctors' office, for instance, M-BUS would fill [get there]. Once a structure is chosen to fill a slot it acts as an independent memory structure. What happened, say, in the car on the way to the office can usually only be reconstructed. That is, we can guess at our normative mode of transportation to professionals' offices and attempt to figure out what might have happened on a particular trip.

The most important aspect of the structures organized by a MOP is that they be general enough to be used by other MOPs. This is a key point. Scenes and scripts organized by one MOP can also be organized by others. For example, the PAY scene is used by a great many MOPs in addition to M-POV. If you lost your wallet you might atempt to figure out where you had it last. You might remember putting it down near a cash register while paying. The problem then would be to differentiate one PAY event from another. The fact that this is difficult indicates that PAY is a shared structure.

There is another way in which sharing memory structures can cause memory confusion. An event that takes place in WAITING ROOM will be stored in WAITING ROOM and thus will be linked to M-POV. But M-POV can be linked to a variety of different situations (doctors, accountants, lawyers, etc.) that use M-POV. Thus, an event that takes place in a WAITING ROOM may easily become disassociated from which particular waiting room was used. A person may be able to recall that the event in question occurred in a waiting room, but think it was the doctor's when actually it was the dentist's.

So the disadvantage of sharing memory structures is that it creates possibilities for memory confusion. This is outweighed, however, by the advantage gained in allowing generalizations. At the cost of being unable, on occasion, to remember what waiting room a certain event occurred in, or where a certain instance of paying took place, we gain the advantage of having all the knowledge we have acquired from all our professional office visits, or from all the situations in which we have had to pay for something, available to us to deal with a new situation.

The sharing of scenes such as PAY complicates the relationship of MOPs to the scripts that frequently occur in them. For example, there are many ways of doing PAY (i.e., there are many methods of payment). These methods are represented by various scripts which can be used to color pay, such as *$CASH REGISTER*, *$BILLING*, etc. The various scripts associated with PAY are organized by PAY in memory. After one particular method of payment takes place, PAY is augmented to contain the information that the event occurred. In the case of payment associated with the doctor visit, two links are added. One says that this event in PAY was part of M-CONTRACT, and one that says that it was part of M-POV. (Actually, more links than this are needed because there are more MOPs active here, but this simplification will do for this example.) These links allow the retrieval of the particular scripts which have been used to color the scene in previous instances of a particular MOP. For instance, this would allow us to recover the fact that in most instances of M-POV, the payment script used is *$BILLING*. Thus the indexing of scripts under scenes allows us to remember variations on general scenes which are specific to a certain MOP, while still retaining the ability to make generalizations based on components of the scene which are common to all occurrences of it.

At the point in understanding when M-POV has been accessed then, we are ready to add new events to the memory structures that M-POV organizes. Further, we can use M-POV to fill in implicit information between steps in a chain of events by assuming that intermediate scenes not explicitly stated actually took place and should be processed. As we have said,

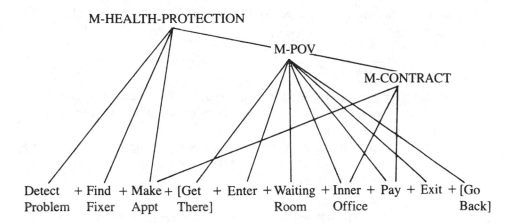

M-HEALTH-PROTECTION

M-POV

M-CONTRACT

Detect + Find + Make + [Get + Enter + Waiting + Inner + Pay + Exit + [Go
Problem   Fixer   Appt   There]   Room   Office   Back]

Figure 2

the first sentence, "I went to the doctor's yesterday," gets us to look at what we know about doctors. Some of what we know are the MOPs that are activated by a visit to a doctor. Thus we activate M-POV and M-CONTRACT as we said before. This allows us to predict generally what sequence of events will follow. Now when the sentence "While I was reading a magazine I noticed that a patient who arrived after me was being taken ahead of me" is encountered, it can be interpreted in terms of knowledge stored in M-POV about WAITING ROOMS. What we have here is an expectation failure from the script of **customer queueing** that is organized by WAITING ROOM. We can understand that there is a potential problem here because of our failed expectation for what normally happens in WAITING ROOM. This expectation was activated by M-POV, which activated WAITING ROOM, which activated $CUSTOMER QUEUE-ING, which held the actual expectation.

The final sentence "The doctor will probably still overcharge me!" refers to the PAY scene of M-CONTRACT.

So, seen all at once, what we have in a "doctor visit" are three MOPs, each of which connects to the various scenes that contain the expectations necessary for processing, and in terms of which memories will be stored. Seen temporally, each scene follows the next, so the end product looks very much like a script (in the old sense). But, we have no reason to believe that any structure that represents such a linear combination of scenes, ever exists in memory as one whole piece at one time (Figure 2).

Actually, there are some other MOPs relevant here too. For example, a trip of sorts is involved in this visit and that is a TRIP MOP. Similarly there are MOPs active for the doctor's motivations and for higher level issues.

Some perspective

We have, to this point, used three different kinds of memory structures in our discussions. What are the general characteristics that these structures share?

Any structure in memory that can be used as both a container of memories and of information relevant to processing new inputs must contain the following things:

> a prototype
> a set of expectations organized in terms of the prototype
> a set of memories organized in terms of the previously failed expectations of the prototype
> a characteristic goal.

A MOP organizes such structures. A scene is a general description of a setting and activities in pursuit of a goal relevant to that setting. A script is a particular instantiation of a scene. Ordinarily, there are many scripts attached to one scene. (That is, a scene that had no scripts tht instantiated it, would not look in any way different from a script, as it would have only one set of expectations about how things would happen.)

Given the above definitions, let us now consider how the memory and understanding process might work. An episode does not enter memory as a unit. Various knowledge sources are used in the processing of any episode. During that processing, those knowledge sources are changed by the information in the episode. What we know about a subject is altered by new information about that subject. Any episode we process provides such new information. Since a new episode carries information of many different types, this implies that the initial episode has been somehow *broken up,* with its various pieces being assigned different locations in memory depending on the knowledge used to process them.

According to this view then, memory would seem to have a set of knowledge structures, each of which contains pieces of various episodes. However, it seems unlikely that this is exactly the case. Under some circumstances when an episode breaks into pieces, each piece is useless in retrieving the other pieces of that episode. At other times, an entire episode is retrievable through a piece of that episode.

This difference is related to the problem of reconstructive memory. Consider an argument that one has with one's spouse in a car. Is it possible to retrieve the purpose or destination of the trip, or what happened prior to entry into the car? The answer depends upon the reconstructability of the episode given a scene from that episode. An episode is reconstructable if there are events or objects present in a scene from that episode that in some sense depend on prior or subsequent scenes. Such dependence can be of two types. The dependence may occur because a particular element is present in the given scene that directly correlates with a specific element in a prior or subsequent scene. Or, the dependence may occur because general information is available by which the prior and subsequent scenes can be *figured out*.

In the latter case, we have an instance of the use of MOPs. MOPs provide, among other things, the temporal precedences among scenes in a standard situation. We know that an airplane trip involves arrival at the airport, followed by checking in, followed by waiting in the waiting area and so on. This information is all part of M-AIRPLANE TRIP.

We can use this information to reconstruct episodes based on the memory of some portion of them. That is, given a scene, by examining a MOP that it might belong to, we can infer what other scenes must also have occurred. When any memory structure is considered as a possible holder of a memory that we are seeking, we can search that structure by using indices that were found in the initial scene. We are claiming, then, that episodes are broken apart in terms of the structures employed in understanding them, stored in terms of those structures in memory, and are reconstructable by various search techniques. Episodes are not remembered as wholes but as pieces.

What are the limits on the range and kinds of structures that MOPs order? Also, what kinds of orderings are there on MOPs?

Using the goal classifications given in Schank and Abelson (1977), we can see that MOPs relate strongly to the achievement of a certain level of goals. There are MOPs that attempt to achieve almost all these goal types. For example:

Satisfaction	S-goal	M-RESTAURANT; M-HOTEL
Enjoyment	E-goal	M-BOWLING; M-THEATER
Achievement	A-goal	***
Preservation	P-goal	M-CONTRACT
Crisis	C-goal	M-FIREDEPT; M-POV
Delta	D-goal	M-LIBRARY; M-BUS
Instrumental	I-goal	M-TRIP; M-SCHOOL; M-WEDDING

One point here is that it is not easy to find clear examples of MOPs that realize achievement goals. A-goals are at a higher level than the other goal types mentioned above. Notions such as M-SUCCESS, M-POWER, or M-REVOLUTION simply do not make sense at the level we have been discussing. MOPs order scenes (where scenes are defined as settings plus relevant scripts) in the service of simple low level goals (where simple low level goals are defined as those listed above, but not A-goals). Since scripts are merely stereotyped plans, MOPs also serve the function of ordering plans. Thus MOPs relate to what we termed *Named Plans* in Schank and Abelson (1977). Further, since plans are intended to realize goals, really what we are doing here is attempting to uncover the elaborate goal classification and organization system used by the mind. In other words, we are suggesting that goals are the basis of memory organization. We remember an event primarily in terms of the goals to which it pertains.

An example

Consider the problem of recalling the details of a particular visit to a city that one has frequently visited. No one structure in memory contains all the details of this trip. There is, however, likely to be a node in memory that contains some of the details of the trip directly and through which much of the trip can be reconstructed. The following things seem to be true:

1. Some details of the trip may be recalled apart from the purpose of the trip.
2. The purpose of the trip may be recalled apart from details of the trip that were not connected with that purpose.
3. Incidents that occurred on the trip that had nothing to do in principle with the trip (i.e., reading a certain book) may be recalled completely apart from the trip (that is, no connection is even available).
4. Scenes normally associated with trips can be reconstructed, but many of their details will be missing.
5. The trip may be recalled through some conclusion or generalization drawn from it at an appropriate time (i.e., "That reminds me of the time I took a trip and had no expectations for it and everything worked out perfectly").
6. The trip may be recalled through some malfunction in the ordinary flow of the trip.
7. The trip may be recalled by any of its scenes being brought to mind.
8. Scenes that were part of one trip may get confused with similar scenes that were part of other trips.
9. Results or effects of the trip may serve as cues for recalling different scenes of the trip.

There are other issues that could be stated here as well, but these will do for now. Anything that can be remembered in its own right, apart from the trip itself, is a candidate for consideration as a structure in memory. Thus, since the purpose of the trip (a meeting say) can be recalled apart from the trip itself, that purpose is a structure. Similarly if the airplane ride can be recalled apart from the trip, there must be a separate structure for it. Additionally, since some structures clearly package other structures in a way as to allow reconstruction, there must be such structures available in memory as well.

Thus, we would expect structures such as M-ATTEND MEETING, M-TRIP, M-AIRPLANE, M-RENT-A-CAR, M-HOTEL to exist. Some of these structures point to others. M-TRIP would include M-AIRPLANE, M-HOTEL, and M-RENT-A-CAR, for example. Within these MOPs would be various scenes such as *check into the hotel, coffee break at meeting,* and so on. Some of these scenes are retrievable through others and some are retrievable only directly. Thus, it might be possible to reconstruct what hotel one stayed in and therefore the *check out* scene by recalling information about the physical surroundings in the *discussion* scene in M-ATTEND MEETING. On the other hand, it is rather unlikely, unless something peculiar occurred there, that the *rent-a-car bus* scene would be easily recalled by anything other than direct search. To recall such a scene it is almost always necessary to get to it via the MOP that it is a part of. In other words, to answer a question such as:

What was the seat configuration in the rent-a-car bus?

it is necessary to go from M-TRIP to M-RENT-A-CAR and then to the right scene, in order to answer the question. There really is no other way to get to that scene. Such information can only be found by finding the one scene that stores those low level details.

Other MOPs, and therefore other scenes, can be related to such a trip, of course. For example, one might also use the structures M-ROMANCE, M-BUSINESS DEAL, or M-PARTY. Further, the juxtaposition of various MOPs and goals associated with those MOPs might cause one to place certain aspects of a particular trip in special structures.

The point is that many things can go on in one's life at one time. A trip to attend a meeting can have an unexpected business deal, a romance, a travel screw up and so on as part of it. These would tend to get disassociated from the original experience because of "mushing" in scenes and reconstruction from scenes. But they do not get forgotten, merely placed in different structures. Each of these things would be remembered in its own structure, disassociated from the particular trip, and involved with others of their kind (i.e., romances with other romances, business deals with other business deals).

The connection in memory between these items can come in either of two places. One possibility is that since they were a part of the flow of events, their place in time can be retrieved in the reconstruction process. This assumes the view that reconstruction in memory means going through a scene, finding what MOP or MOPs it was part of, and then searching other scenes organized by that MOP with indices derived from the original scene.

The other possibility is that a TOP has been created for them. A TOP is a high level structure in memory that stores information independent from any particular domain. TOPs represent generalizations or conclusions having to do with abstractions from actual events. The plot of Romeo and Juliet would be stored in terms of a TOP about mutual goal pursuit. Similarly, a belief that *happenstance business deals result from trips whose main purpose is a meeting of another sort* might be stored in terms of some *fortuitous circumstances* TOP. TOPs will be discussed in Chapter 7.

Memory then, is a morass of complex structures, related by the episodes they point to and the temporal and causal connections between them. Our task is to sort out the morass by identifying the place and purpose of a set of memory structures that would account for various memory phenomena.

6   MOPs

Scenes

A MOP is an orderer of scenes. To better see how MOPs function therefore, it is necessary to have a good grasp of what a scene is. A simple
definition of a scene is:

A memory structure that groups together actions with a shared goal, that occurred at the same time. It provides a sequence of general actions. Specific
memories are stored in scenes, indexed with respect to how they differ from the
general action in the scene.

The above definition needs some more fleshing out, and we shall provide that shortly, but it will do for now.

Scenes organize specific memories in terms of their relationship to the
general structure of that scene. MOPs do not explicitly contain memories.
Rather, they organize scenes that contain memories. Scripts represent
common instantiations of a scene. Thus, a scene consists of a generally-
defined sequence of actions, whereas a script represents particular realizations of the generalizations in a scene. Specific memories can be organized under scripts, in terms of expectation failures. This follows from the
above, since a script is no more than a scene that has been colored
(particularly instantiated) in a given way.

The scenes we have discussed in previous chapters relied upon physical
settings for their basis. We left *setting information* out of the definition of
a scene given above, because, as we shall see, some scenes are not physically defined. Goals are a better candidate for centrality in the base
memory structure, given their significance in memory. Yet setting seems
to be intrinsic to the nature of many of the scenes we have discussed so
far. We call such scenes *physical scenes:*

A physical scene is a scene that has a physical setting as its common thread. Thus,
put all together, a physical scene has a setting, delimited by the range of one's

95

visual field, a defining goal, and a common time, all of which contribute to delimiting and packaging a set of actions.

Most of the scenes we have used so far are physical scenes. They represent a kind of *snapshot* of one's surroundings at a given time. Memories grouped in physical scenes provide information about what happened and how things looked. But not everthing we know and care about is physical. Ordering of memories can occur if the memories are made up of information that is not physical in its basis. Thus, for example, we can know something about how an event can manifest itself societally. This is the essence of M-CONTRACT, the MOP that we mentioned earlier as a part of a doctor visit.

M-CONTRACT organizes some scenes that are not physically bounded. Entities such as AGREE, or DELIVER, while behaving very much like scenes in a physcal MOP, have no specific physical instantiation. They can happen anywhere and can take a great many different physical forms. Nevertheless, M-CONTRACT is a MOP. It functions in every way like M-POV. It points to an ordered set of scenes. These scenes are the holders of memories indexed in terms of expectations that have failed. Thus, a failure to deliver agreed-upon services will be indexed under the DELIVER scene in M-CONTRACT. In this way, a failure of a department store to deliver a package that was paid for might remind one of a restaurant that required pre-payment and then failed to serve the desired food. Such reminding can only be accounted for by a memory organization that has scenes that are not exclusively physically bounded. That is, there are also *societal scenes:*

Societal scene definition

A societal scene is a scene that has a social setting as its common thread. A social setting is defined as a social relationship that obtains between two people for some particular purpose. Thus, a societal scene has a social setting that involves two people, each pursuing a goal that the other person is a necessary participant in, at a common time, with a communication link between them. The actions comprising the interaction between the participants defines the scene.

A societal scene, then, expresses a generalization about how people will interact in some socially-defined situation. But how can the boundaries of a socially-defined situation be established? For example, a restaurant or a doctor's office can be viewed as one large social situation or a set of smaller ones. Any decomposition into a set of scenes has potential payoff from the point of view of learning and generalization. What makes *restaurant* and *doctor's office visit* too large to be one scene is that they contain multiple interactions between people for different low-level goals.

Thus, the defining characteristic of a societal scene is that it is organized around the pursuit of a single goal by one of the characters in it.

The third and last kind of scene is what we call the **personal scene.** It is responsible for idiosyncratic behavior that is personally defined:

A personal scene is a scene whose common thread is a particular goal that belongs to the person whose scene it is. Any private plan to achieve one's own ends that is liable to repeat itself frequently is a possible personal scene. Settings, both physical and social, may or may not enter into personal scenes. There can be no more than one setting and one time per scene. Personal scenes are heavily idiosyncratic. They form one's private plans to achieve goals.

MOPs defined

We are now ready to define a MOP:

A MOP consists of a set of scenes directed towards the achievement of a goal. A MOP always has one major scene whose goal is the essence or purpose of the events organized by the MOP.

Since memories are to be found in scenes, a very important part of memory organization is our ability to travel from scene to scene. A MOP is an organizer of scenes. Finding the appropriate MOP, in memory search, enables one to answer the question, "What would come next?" where the answer is another scene. That is, MOPs provide information about how various scenes are connected to one another.

The distinction we made at the scene level creates a parallel distinction in MOPs. Most of the MOPs we have discussed so far have been **Physical MOPs.** Physical MOPs can contain scenes that seem societal in nature, but what is actually happening is that one event is being governed by two scenes. Thus, for example, both M-CONTRACT which is a *Societal MOP*, and M-AIRPLANE, which is physical, share a PAY scene. But each relates to different aspects of that event. In other words, *paying* can be seen as both a physical event and also as a societal event. Different MOPs provide expectations in each case. Events confirming those expectations will be remembered in terms of both of the scenes that were active.

Personal MOPs are idiosyncratic sets of scenes that can include both personal scenes and either physical or societal scenes. To some extent, all MOPs are idiosyncratic of course. Personal MOPs have the added feature that they may have no relation to how someone else might behave. Thus, we may have our own way of pursuing goals on a date with a member of the opposite sex, that bear no relationship to the way anyone else behaves. Any planned behavior that is entirely self-motivated and self-initiated, without regard to how others may make plans for similar goals, would be encoded in a personal MOP. Some personal MOPs can be a variation on a more standard MOP, where some personal scenes are added to, or replace, one or more standard physical or societal scenes. It is also possible to have personal MOPs that are made up exclusively of personal scenes. These might relate to one's own particular way of getting what one wants. Personal MOPs are goal-driven, as are other MOPs, but they tend to be used in pursuit of higher level goals than the others. For very high level goals, even personal MOPs can become relatively standardized. Thus, health preservation for example, would relate to a personal MOP for dealing with this goal that might be quite a bit like everyone else's method. The important point in personal MOPs is how they are related to high level goals. People tend to be more idiosyncratic in pursuing high-level goals than in pursuing mundane ones. As a result, personal MOPs tend to be those which relate to high-level goal pursuit.

Since nearly every episode has a physical, societal, and personal aspect to it, any episode is likely to have at least three different MOPs that are useful in processing what goes on in it. These same three MOPs will also be used for storing the memories that result from that processing. To put this another way, when a person visits a doctor, his visit can be understood, stored, and later recalled, in terms of its physical aspects – driving, waiting, being examined, leaving, etc. It can also be understood in terms of its societal aspects, in this case an implicit agreement to pay for services rendered. In addition, the visit can be understood in terms of the various goals that were being operated on by the participants in the events. In the patients's case this is M-HEALTH PRESERVATION. In the doctor's, M-JOB controls the action. These personal aspects of an event also serve in the processing of the event. Further, we would expect that attempts to preserve one's health would be stored with similar attempts in one's memory. If this were not the case, it would be very difficult to learn from past experience about what to do when there is a health problem. Similarly, we expect the doctor to store job related events together with other events similarly characterized.

The above three-part division is relevant for processing any input event. Put another way, we are suggesting that for every input, one must ask the following questions:

> What transpired physically?
> Where did those events take place?
>
> What societal conventions were employed?
> What impact did the events have on the social position of the participants?
>
> What personal effect occurred on the participants?
> What personal goals were achieved by the events?

Each pair of questions corresponds to one kind of scene (and MOP) that is used in processing an event.

Meta-MOPs

The MOPs we have been describing are based on sequences of scenes organized around an object and its role in the world. That is, MOPs such as DOCTOR, AIRPLANE, or MUSEUM are simply stereotypical objects or settings that are used in a stereotypical sequence of events. Further, their use implies a set of scenes that naturally precede and follow them. Thus, these MOPs bear a strong similarity to our old definition of scripts. They are stereotypical sequences of socially-defined patterns. What other kinds of MOPs might there be?

In Schank and Abelson (1977), we suggested that information about planning was organized in entities that we called NAMED PLANS. These entities consisted of units conjoined in the way that MOPs are conjoined. Thus, we had:

USE (X) = D-KNOW (LOC(X)) + D-PROX + D-CONT + I-PREP + DO

This meant that a plan to use something (X) was made up of steps, namely: finding out where X is; getting in contact with X; gaining control of X; do some preparatory steps defined by the nature of X; and then doing what one had in mind in the first place.

Is a named plan another kind of MOP? Or, is it right at all? Certainly, there is a sense in which this sort of structure is appropriate. But, if this is a MOP, then it is a new kind of MOP, because it does not organize scenes based in physical settings. Rather, it organizes entities that organize scenes. Thus, it is a kind of template by which MOPs in general are constructed. We call this entity a *meta-MOP*.

In the last chapter we referred to M-TRIP. It is more likely that TRIP is a meta-MOP, so we will now designate it mM-TRIP. The distinction between a MOP and a meta-MOP is not all that hard. We are simply noting that MOPs organize scenes, whereas a structure that organizes MOPs is somewhat different. Actually, it is not all that different. There really is a continuum here. To find memories, as we have said, it is necessary to find scenes. A MOP can point out what scenes might be relevant. A meta-MOP points out entities at a higher level than a scene. Particular MOPs then change such generalized scenes into the more familiar scenes that we have been using. (Generalized scenes are discussed in Chapter 9.) As we shall see later on, the difference here depends upon the experience of the individual whose memory structures these are.

A trip can be described very generally as:

> mm-TRIP = PLAN + GET RESOURCES + MAKE ARRANGE-
> MENTS + PREPARATORY TRAVEL + PREPARATION
> + PRIMARY TRAVEL + ARRIVAL + DO

This is a meta-MOP which can be used to reconstruct MOPs that organize scenes that conform to its pattern. Thus it can be used to construct M-AIRPLANE which looks as follows:

> M-AIRPLANE = PLAN + GET MONEY + CALL AIRLINE
> + GET TICKETS + DRIVE TO AIRPORT + CHECK IN
> + WAITING AREA + BOARDING + FLYING
> + DEPLANING. . . .]

There is a natural progression of structures that we have discussed so far that suggests itself:

> meta MOPs
> MOPs
> scenes
> scripts

Meta MOPs describe ordered progressions of abstract generalized scenes. As such they provide the stuff out of which MOPs are made. They do not actually contain memories. MOPs are more specific descriptions of such progressions. They contain actual scenes, which in turn contain specific memories.

Processing with MOPs

When we begin to specify what MOPs will be used in processing a specific story, the question arises: what can be a MOP? How many MOPs are there likely to be in a system? Is their number or range fixed?

These same questions necessarily arise in the course of research on scripts and schemata. It has seemed plausible for researchers in this area to answer questions about how a sentence concerning subject X is processed with something like the **X script** or the **X schema.** Such an answer implies that any body of knowledge can be a script (or schema). But, if the range of knowledge structures that are potentially used is too large, the problem of deciding upon the correct structure at a given time can be overwhelming.

As we have said, storing all the knowledge one has about X in one chunk prohibits generalization between experiences with X and related ones with Y and Z. With MOPs, the issue of what structures there can be in a system becomes a question of how general a high level knowledge structure can be in its storage of information. If we store things generally, then useful generalization can occur across contexts. Thus we can learn from experiences across contexts. But, if we store information too generally, we will fail to develop specialized knowledge of the kind that illustrates expertise. Expertise is nice of course, but it can overload a system if there is too much expertise available at the same time. Thus it is the performance of the system as a whole which provides the constraint on what MOPs there can be.

There can be no correct answer to what kind of content a MOP can have and therefore to what is and is not a MOP. Any prototype that provides expectations can be a knowledge structure in memory. When an ordering of structures is observed to hold, then a MOP exists. In other words, MOPs and structures are viewpoints imposed by an observer on the world. A person can (perhaps tentatively) believe that the world has a certain structure. This belief will cause expectations to arise about what will happen next. Memories will be indexed in terms of failures obtained from those expectations. Prototypes will be developed that indicate what entities are expected. In other words, memory creates its own organization. An organization is not imposed upon people or their memories.

Having said this, we can begin to discuss what particular structures and MOPs might be present in a typical observer of the world. Whatever claims we make about which MOPs and which structures are necessary for processing a particular story are not immutable. It helps, since the world is not entirely chaotic, to have structures and MOPs in one's memory that relate to the rest of the world's collective view of the world. But no one person's view is the same as any other person's view. The more one knows about a subject, the more one must change one's view of that subject. So, the more one knows about a subject, the more one's MOPs and structures for processing information about that subject differ from the rest of the world's collective view of that subject.

Let us consider the processing of a hypothetical news story that describes a diplomatic visit for the purpose of negotiations. The story begins: "Cyrus Vance has gone on a trip to Israel to negotiate with Menachem Begin." After we have read this sentence, we are prepared for a great many different kinds of information. Depending upon what we already know about Cyrus Vance, negotiations, plane trips, the Middle East, and so on, we must be prepared to use that knowledge in order to understand what we are being told. In this sense, understanding has two main parts. First, we must be able to infer things we are not told directly. Second, we must be able to fit what we are told and what we have inferred into an overall picture of what is going on. In other words, we must update what we know. To do each of these we must be prepared to process what we have not yet seen. This helps us eliminate ambiguities and enables us to pay more processing attention to the unexpected, where it is needed most. To summarize, in our view understanding consists of:

1. Creation of expectations
2. Inference of implicit information
3. Memory modification (learning)

Any memory structures we propose for handling a simple story about Cyrus Vance's trip to Israel must be useful for the above tasks. To put this more concretely, whatever we might want to know about this trip must have a place to go in memory once we know it. Further, whatever implicit information we wish to glean from what we hear must have been present explicitly in a memory structure that was accessed during processing. We are asking then: What information and memories do we need? In what memory structures are they to be found? How do we access them at just the right time?

Some memory structures that might be active here are given below. (Note that the structures in Vance's head would normally be different from those in an observer's head. Those listed below are just some hypothetical ones that are supposed to reflect Vance's structures.)

(PHYSICAL)	(SOCIETAL)	(PERSONAL)
M-AIRPLANE	M-TREATY	M-CONVINCE
	-SIGNING	-PERSON
M-MEETING	M-CONTRACT	M-PATRIOTISM
M-STATE DINNER	M-FRIENDSHIP	M-ACT-IN-ROLE

The memory structures alluded to above are intended to be illustrative of some of the kinds of knowledge that apply to understanding this situation. Many of the above MOPs may apply at the same time. That is, they may each provide expectations with respect to any given action. They may relate to, or share, given scenes, although MOPs of different types would relate to different realizations of the events. Thus, a meeting for the purposes of negotiation in which each participant was trying to defend the interests of his country would require at least one MOP of each type to help in processing. When Vance stands up at a critical moment in negotiating, it can be seen as a physical act (he got up to go somewhere); a societal act (he wanted to indicate his disgust with the proposals; he wanted to indicate that the United States is not easily pushed around); or a personal act (he felt like he couldn't take it any more; he had to go to the bathroom). Different MOPs provide various expectations here so that these interpretations can be made at any given point.

Having said that, let us look at Vance's trip to Israel a bit more carefully. From a physical point of view, certain things happened on the trip. Whatever else this story is, it is also a story about an airplane trip. In order to have that knowledge available for use, we must have recognized this fact (and all the other structures that this story is an instance of must be similarly recognized). An event that takes place in an airplane can be recalled by remembering the physical aspects of the situation. Understanding that an airplane was used for transportation may or may not turn out to be important in understanding what went on. Information about airplanes must be accessed for understanding this story. Further, we can expect that anything we are told about the airplane part of the trip would use memories from the M-AIRPLANE to help us in understanding it. Expectation failures from M-AIRPLANE would be stored in M-AIRPLANE. Events that occurred in the airplane, say an important discussion with an aide, would likely be stored some place in memory other than M-AIR-PLANE. In that case M-AIRPLANE would simply be background, not of great use for retrieval.

How do we know to access M-AIRPLANE? This same question can be asked about any of the MOPs. How do we know which memory structures that will be useful in understanding a trip? This is where meta-MOPs play their part. The meta-MOP mM-TRIP tells us that a trip is usually comprised of a set of structures that occur in a certain order. It also tells us what structures are likely to fill those slots and under what conditions. Thus mM-TRIP looks roughly like this:

> [make arrangements] + |*[get to main transport] + [do preparations for main transport] + [do main transport] + [welcome] + [get from main transport]*|+ {do business} + {sleeping arrangements} + [rerun inner loop bounded by |* *|]

In addition, mM-TRIP tells us that long trips require airplanes, that officials of the United States are likely to fly special planes from Air Force bases, and so on.

The role of a meta-MOP then is to point to structures in memory that are likely to be relevant (if we are processing) or to have been relevant (if we are attempting to retrieve information). Thus, mM-TRIP points to M-CAR which contains what we know about driving someplace. It also points to M-LIMOUSINE. Both of these structures will fill the placeholder **[get to main transport]** in mM-TRIP. Knowing that Vance lost an umbrella on the trip, and knowing that Cyrus Vance usually gets driven by limousine to airports, allows us to consider searching M-LIMOUSINE to see if we remember him having it there. Knowing where to search is one of the major problems of retrieval in memory. It is the role of meta-MOPs to point to the MOPs that are likely to have been active in the original processing of a situation and hence are likely to contain the memories of that situation.

Meta-MOPs also play a role in the explanation of people's behavior. We are always attempting to find out why a character is doing what he is doing. The answer to why someone is doing a given action can be on many levels. A person's behavior can be explained by reference to themes that are active in his life for example (Schank & Abelson, 1977). We can understand why someone is doing something in terms of the higher level goals that his actions are an attempt to achieve. But, we can also satisfy ourselves with lower level explanations that refer only to the role of an action in some plan. To answer, "Why did Vance get in his limousine?" with "to get to the airport, to take a plane . . ." is to give a rather low level explanation for his actions. Nevertheless, we do look for such explanations so we can fit in a set of actions within an overall plan. Meta-MOPs provide these explanations.

MOPs and scripts

We have alluded several times in the course of defining MOPs to the relationship between MOPs and the version of scripts as presented in Schank and Abelson (1977). We have done so because we believe the question of how they relate is both an obvious and important one. Before we leave the subject of MOPs (temporarily) we would like to examine this issue once more in detail.

The question may be put: If MOPs are things like M-AIRPLANE and M-STATE, DINNER, what have we really done that is different from our work on scripts? Have we just replaced a $ with an M?

One of our initial motivations for revamping our theory of high level knowledge structures was to account for the possibility of recognition confusions in memory. We were also dissatisfied with several of the scripts used by SAM, for example $ACCIDENT. We were looking for psychologically valid high level structures that could be used for both processing and storage. We wanted appropriate remindings to be accounted for by whatever structures we proposed.

What is the difference between $AIRPLANE and M-AIRPLANE?

The difference between MOPs and scripts:
A MOP is an ordered set of scenes.
A script (1977 version) is an ordered set of scenes.
BUT – The definition of scene is different in each case.

For a MOP, a scene is a structure that can be shared by a great many other MOPs. For a script (1977 version) a scene was particular to a given script and was not accessible without using that script.

A script (new version) is scene-specific. No script transcends the boundaries of a scene.

Now, to make this specific, let us actually look at M-AIRPLANE and *$AIRPLANE*. *$AIRPLANE* (that is, the 1977 version of that script) was more or less a list of all the events of an entire airplane trip. It included making the reservation, getting to the airport, checking in, riding in the plane, eating the meal and so on. In SAM and FRUMP these would all be things stored in a single complex structure, complete with optional tracks, under the name *$AIRPLANE*.

However, such a structure is useless for generalization or reminding across contexts and within contexts. For this, we need structures that are far more general than a detailed list of events, however complex. For example, getting someplace by car, and making reservations by telephone, are two scenes that would necessarily be part of *$AIRPLANE* that could not possibly be part of M-AIRPLANE. The reason for this is that one could easily confuse one trip in a car to visit a friend who lives near the airport with a trip to the airport that was intended to enable one to fly someplace. Similarly, one could easily confuse a phone conversation making airline reservations with one making hotel reservations. In fact they might well be the same conversation.

The problem with our old conception of scripts was that much too much that could have been defined generally, and that is likely to be stored in a general fashion in memory, was defined specifically as a part of a particular script. When one takes away from *$AIRPLANE* everything that could have been defined generally, one is left with the things specific to *$AIRPLANE,* namely getting on the plane, being seated, being instructed about oxygen masks, and so on. These are what we now call scripts. That is, M-AIRPLANE as a MOP, organizes a set of scenes. One of these scenes is CHECK IN. But, CHECK IN is a scene that is shared by a great many MOPs. (For example, M-DOCTOR VISIT and M-HOTEL might also use CHECK IN.) So, various specializations of CHECK IN exist that supply detailed knowledge that colors the generality of that scene. Thus, *$AIRPLANE CHECK IN* is a script that is attached to CHECK IN that gets used, in conjunction with the generalizations available from CHECK IN itself, when M-AIRPLANE is active. (The structure of scripts such as *$AIRPLANE CHECK IN* also differs from the old notion of a script in its failure-driven organization, as we have described. Thus, experiences that occur within them, while those scripts are directing processing, that do not coincide with the expectations generated by that script, are to be encoded as failures and indexed within that script.)

This leaves us with a rather impoverished airplane script, but with a much more powerful memory organization. Much of what was in $AIR-PLANE is now in mM-TRIP. Making reservations, getting to the plane and so on, are handled by MOPs activated by mM-TRIP. M-AIRPLANE fills one placeholder of mM-TRIP, the one we labeled [do main transport] above. It consists of the following scenes:

> M-AIRPLANE's scenes
> CHECK-IN + WAITING AREA + BOARDING
>   + SIT-IN-THE-PLANE + DEPLANE + COLLECT-BAGS

Each of the scenes used by M-AIRPLANE is constructed as generally as possible. However, the idiosyncratic history of a given person's memory makes its presence felt here. For example, above we listed as one of the scenes of M-AIRPLANE, something called WAITING AREA. Now it is reasonable to ask, is this the same as the scene we called WAITING ROOM in M-POV? Clearly, the answer to such a question depends upon the experiences a person has had and the generalizations that person has formulated. It is perfectly plausible that a person who had been to a doctor's and a lawyer's office and had constructed a scene WAITING ROOM, might upon his first encounter with an airport, see the waiting area as a version of WAITING ROOM. And, of course, he might not.

Our point is that the possibility for such generalizations, for interpreting a new experience in terms of what it believes to be its most relevant old one, must exist for a memory. In order to do this, scenes must be memory structures in their own right, distinct from the structures they are used with in processing. Scripts, in the 1977 version, were too restrictive in this regard. This does not mean that scripts do not exist. Some of the experimental work on scripts relates to MOPs as we have now defined them and some of it relates to our new, more restricted definition of scripts.

One problem is, given a memory with MOPs, scenes, scripts, and other structures, we might assume that we have a set of immutable entities with no flexibility. The most interesting facet of human memory is our ability to take an input and find the most relevant memory we have to help process it. This is done by a reliance on indices derived from expectation failures. In essence, failure is the root of change. Thus, memory adapts successfully by failing often. But one practical problem for a theorist here, is that since the memory structures we propose are so changeable, we will have trouble making definite statements about their specifics.

Thus, the issue of what can be a scene or a MOP must await a description of the processes by which memory alters its existing structures. There is no right answer to what can be a scene or a MOP. The actual entities used by a memory vary according to the inputs that have been processed and the generalizations that have been made.

What we can do here is discuss the nature of structures that are likely to be active in an example; so let us return to the question of what we need to process our story about Cyrus Vance. Recall that for any input about a person we must ask physical, societal and personal questions in order to access the requisite MOPs. For this story the physical MOPs needed include:

meta-MOPs	MOPs
mM-TRIP	M-AIRPLANE
	M-HOTEL
	M-MEETING
	M-STATE DINNER

Listing all of the scenes that these MOPs organize would be rather pointless, but it is nevertheless important to get a feel for their level of generality. For example, the scene CHECK-IN is used by both M-AIRPLANE and M-HOTEL. This, of course, can create confusions in recall, but, as we have said, such confusions are the price we pay for learning by generalization. Both M-MEETING and M-AIRPLANE have a strand for [get to place]. This strand is likely to be filled in both cases by the scene DRIVE. Similarly each has the potential scene GREETING after DRIVE is over. The fact that GREETING is optional and frequently absent will nevertheless not ameliorate potential confusions, such as trying to recall where an odd thing that happened while you were being introduced to somebody actually occurred.

The societal MOPs that are likely to be active for this story are:

meta-MOPs	MOPs
mM-NEGOTIATE	M-MEETING
	M-DISCUSSION
	M-CONTRACT
mM-DIPLOMACY	M-FRIENDSHIP
	M-SOCIAL-OCCASION

This is not intended to be an exhaustive list for this story. We are simply trying to give the flavor of the kinds of structures that it might be necessary to employ here. Note that many of the MOPs listed above are not exclusively concerned with a diplomatic trip. For example, consider that mM-NEGOTIATE can also be used to understand a story about a labor relations expert whose job it is to negotiate between labor and management. Is it reasonable that such structures be similar or possibly identical? Is there some reason to have wars and strikes grouped similarly in memory? The answer should be obvious. In a case where the memory was that of a negotiator with expertise in one area, if he were called upon to function in the other area, he would of course rely upon his expertise in the first domain to help him in the second. As he became proficient in the second area, he might learn to refine his conceptions of the two related experiences by noting expectation failures, and eventually constructing different structures for each. To take another example, also in the list above, is M-CONTRACT, which was previously used in our dentist story.

The idea is to use all the relevant MOPs we can find, at the right level of generality, and then *color* them with scripts when such knowledge is available. Thus, if we know that mM-TRIP and mM-VIPVISIT are both applicable, we can determine that after the plane lands there may be a red carpet and a speech at the airport. We know that [get to place] will likely be filled by a limousine provided by one of the governments involved, and so on.

Thus determining what is likely to happen next is a matter of first determining what MOPs might be active. Then we must decide what level of description of the episode we are interested in. Do we want to know what will happen next at a physical or at a societal level? Usually we wish to know both. Then we must attempt to mix the MOPs we have collected to create specific expectations relevant to the given situation. After an input appears, we must determine which MOPs it relates to and how that input should affect those MOPs. Every input has the potential for changing the MOPs active in processing it if an expectations violation is detected.

The last set of MOPs active in this story are personal:

meta-MOPs	MOPs
mM-CAREER	M-DIPLOMAT
	M-STATUS
	M-ACT-IN-ROLE
	M-PATRIOTISM
	M-DO-GOOD-JOB
	M-SUCCESS
mM-PERSONAL RELATIONS	M-CONVINCE-PERSON
	M-SEDUCTION

Here we have a view of some of the personal MOPs a diplomat might have. Ignoring most of the details, the point I wish to emphasize is that many different MOPs are potentially active at any given point. Which

MOPs are actually used depends upon the personal goals and habits of the particular participants. In order to understand what someone is doing, we must attempt to assess why they are doing it. Further, doing something requires knowing how to go about it. Personal MOPs serve to codify one's experiences in achieving one's personal goals.

One problem here is that whereas in the case of physical and societal MOPs we were accessing structures that we can reasonably assume are common to many people, personal MOPs present a different situation.

There are a great many different personal world views, and thus in attempting to understand someone's personal MOPs, we are usually in a position of guessing. For that reason, we will not spend too much time on personal MOPs. It helps to know, of course, that one of the MOPs that is operating in the story – M-HEALTH PRESERVATION – is operating in the dentist story. But, speculating on why Cyrus Vance does what he does may be just too difficult for an understander. In a sense, we cannot fully understand somebody until we know what their personal MOPs are. For most people, we never do learn what they are.

Summary

To sum up: There are three levels at which MOPs can occur: physical, societal, and personal. The apparatus used at each of these levels consists of:

1.   meta MOPs that organize MOPs
2.   MOPs that organize scenes
3.   Scenes (that may have scripts attached to them) that organize memories

These structures are what is used to represent domain-dependent knowledge. However, people have knowledge that is independent of particular domains. Structures to handle that knowledge will be discussed next.

7   TOPs

What is a TOP?

A great deal of our ability to understand and of our ability to be creative and novel in our understanding is due to our ability to see connections between events and to draw parallels between events. Of course, when the parallels drawn are between one episode of eating in a restaurant and another similar episode, the sense of creativity in understanding is severely limited. But frequently we draw parallels at a higher level. We see how events in one context are like those in a very different context. We recognize that what we have learned to do in one situation applies in another. We draw conclusions about our own behavior, and that of others, from repeated experiences in different surroundings.

In essence, we are dealing with the problem of learning, learning of a fairly specific kind. When a person acts stupidly in one situation and suffers the consequences, we expect him to learn from his experiences. We find it hard to understand why he would repeat the same behavior in a new, but similar circumstance. The kind of learning from experience we expect of people comes from our belief that people can and do recognize similarities in situations. In other words, what we learn about behavior in restaurants may well be applicable to more than just restaurants. Our experiences in dealing with waitresses may affect how we react in a job interview. Not everything that occurs in a restaurant should be classified in terms of restaurants.

We have used that argument in previous chapters as a justification for structures like MOPs. But even MOPs are too specific. As we noted in Chapter 4, we get reminded across situations that have only very little in common on the surface. Thus, there must be structures that capture similarities between situations that occur in different domains. If we know something about an abstract situation apart from any specific context, that information must reside somewhere in memory.

110

The key to reminding, memory organization and generalization is the ability to create new structures that coordinate or emphasize the abstract significance of a combination of episodes. Structures that represent this abstract, domain-independent, information we call Thematic Organization Points or TOPs. TOPs are responsible for our ability to:

1. Get reminded of a story that illustrates a point.
2. Come up with adages such as, "A stitch in time saves nine" or "Neither a borrower nor a lender be" at an appropriate point.
3. Recognize an old story in new trappings.
4. Notice co-occurrences of seemingly disparate events and draw conclusions from their co-occurrence.
5. *Know* how something will turn out because the steps leading to it have been *seen* before.
6. Learn information from one situation that will apply in another.
7. Predict an outcome for a newly encountered situation.

The first problem to be addressed is the nature of a TOP. We have, until this point, seen three TOPs. They were presented in Chapter 4 as illustrations used for Outcome-Driven Reminding. They were:

PG;EI – Possession Goal; Evil Intent
MG;OO – Mutual Goal; Outside Opposition
AS;UP – Achieve Success; Utilize Power

How do we recognize that a TOP is relevant at any given point? We cannot just create entities ad infinitum, without some belief that these entities can naturally be found in memory at just the right time in processing.

As an example of this consider the concept of *imperialism*. It makes sense to believe that there must be some high level structure in memory that corresponds to the notion of imperialism. The arguments for this are straightforward. People know things about imperialism. They can recognize from a sequence of actions that imperialism is taking place. They have a set of beliefs about what should be done about imperialism, their attitudes toward it and so on.

However, all of this does not argue that there is a TOP devoted to international imperialism. Imagine a situation in which an executive in a large company decides that the particular employees under his control need more office space. He *borrows* offices nearby that are part of his company's set of offices. It is possible that some people in his company but in a different group might resent his intrusion. They might cite previous instances where he *borrowed* offices that later came under his permanent control. He might be accused of being *imperialistic* with respect to office space.

The point is that imperialism is a concept which in its broadest version should be embodied in a TOP structure. If a tighter definition of imperialism (only in international affairs) is used as a TOP, the ability to apply information learned about imperialism to analogous situations would be lost. Ideally, information about political imperialism between countries would be found within this broader TOP indexed by attributes involving countries, land possession, and so on.

One of the most obvious facts about any high level memory structure is that in order to find a given structure, that structure must bear some relationship to the entities that a processing system is already tracking. Thus, TOPs must conform in some way to things we are already looking for while understanding. To take a concrete example, consider the notion of *Escalating Demands*. Such a TOP could have been proposed to handle the Munich/Afghanistan example presented in Chapter 4. But how would we ever find such a TOP? To do so would require that we be tracking demands while processing the story. However, unless we believe that demands are *always* tracked during understanding, it is hard to explain why we would be tracking them here unless we already knew that demands were relevant to the TOP we were trying to find. Thus, to propose a TOP which is indexed by concepts that we were not already tracking during normal understanding would be circular.

The same is true of *imperialism*. If we knew we had to look for imperialism, then we could find it, but knowing we have to look for it is the crux of the problem. As we argued, a structure representing a more general notion of imperialism is of more use. Now, the interesting point is that a more general structure is also easier to call up during processing.

The frame selection problem has concerned everyone investigating frame-based systems (refs). One of the paradoxes that makes it a problem is that one has to be looking for the appropriate frame without knowing that one is looking for it. If one knows one is looking for it, because one looks for it in everything, there will be an awful lot of wasted processing going on. On the other hand, the rules for deciding on the basis of the input that one is in a restaurant or supermarket are obscure, as Charniak (1977) points out.

The solution to both of these problems depends upon high level structures in memory being coded in terms of notions that are already being tracked. With respect to TOPs, this translates into having TOPs formulated in terms of goals, plans, themes, and other entities which must be tracked during the normal understanding process.

The three TOPs that we have already presented (MG;OO, PG;EI, and AS;UP) all fit in with this view of the nature of TOPs. We are proposing

that what we have is sort of a giant road map of goal and plan relationships. We are constantly looking for goals. When we see that someone
has a goal, we head down the road indicated by that goal. As soon as we
hear more about that goal – for example, if we hear about a plan, a
complicating circumstance, a result, or other extra information – that information serves to point us to a particular set of minor roads off the
major road indicated by the initial goal conditions.

When the end of the minor road has been reached, a TOP has been
found. That TOP is the collection of all memories that previously used
that road to get there, that is, ones that had the same goals and conditions. Since there are likely to be a great many memories stored in a TOP,
various indices are needed within the TOP to find particular memories.
Thus, TOPs are convenient collections of memories involving goals and
plans, written in terms of a sufficiently abstract vocabulary to be useful
across domains. In order for cross-contextual reminding to occur, it
should be enough for two situations to share initial goals, planning or
other conditions, and one or more distinguishing features for one to elicit
the other in memory.

Once a TOP is found that is relevant, and reminding occurs, TOPs (like
all memory structures) can be altered by noting unsuccessful outcomes.
Within a TOP, modifications to plans can be placed so as to alter future
decisions about courses of action appropriate to achieve the goal that is
the basis of the TOP.

The range of TOPs

For any reminding experience that crosses contexts, we can expect that
the two experiences shared a goal type, some planning or other conditions, and one or more low level identical features. The first two make up
the TOP, and the features serve as indices within the TOP. Such an analysis holds up with respect to the examples of cross-contextual reminding
we discussed in Chapter 4:

REMINDING	GOAL	CONDITIONS	FEATURES
R&J/West Side Story	Mutual goal pursuit	Outside opposition	Young lovers; false report of death
R&J/Back Street	Mutual goal pursuit	Outside opposition	Explanation: next time inform coplanner

REMINDING	GOAL	CONDITIONS	FEATURES
Munich/ Afghanistan	Possession goal	Evil intent	Countries; invasions
Nixon/ Mayor of New Haven	Achieve power position	Presence of enemies	Political office; campaign promises

As another example of how this all works, consider the example discussed by Norman and Schank (1982):

We were walking on the cliffs about 100 feet over the beach. As we passed a relatively deserted section of the beach, we looked down and saw a man sunbathing, lying naked on the ledge. He was peering out over the beach, looking quite content.

N: Look at that person. I'll bet he's thinking he is hiding from everyone, but he doesn't realize that people above him can see him quite distinctly. He remindes me of an ostrich. Ostrich. Why does it remind me of an ostrich?

Analyzed according to the method given above, for this example we have:

REMINDING	GOAL	CONDITIONS	FEATURES
Sunbather/ ostrich	Goal blocked	Planner unaware	Sand; hiding

We can see from this example and from the others given above, that TOPs are goal-based. Memories are indexed off of TOPs by whatever features happen to be peculiar to those memories. This can range from common explanations and conclusions to simple things like *sand*. Usually, as we have seen, more than one such identical feature is required for one memory to elicit another. Actually, considering that the goal type and conditions would also be identicial in a TOP-based reminding, there really is a great deal of commonality between any two memories stored in a TOP with identical features. These memories share gross characteristics in terms of their goal relationships and conditions, and very particular characteristics that uniquely define those actual memories.

We must ask at this point then about the range of possible TOPs. Can every possible combination of goal and conditions form a TOP? The answer to this is basically *yes*. But, the situation isn't all that bad. The memory we are proposing is self-organizing. That is, we expect that any category that is useful for structuring memories will be used. One that contains too many memories or too few memories will be further discriminated or abandoned as is deemed useful by the memory itself. The consequence of this is that any categorization procedure we propose for a computer memory will undoubtedly reorganize itself given its needs. Lebowitz (1980) and Kolodner (1980) have already made initial attempts at constructing such memories.

It follows that any organization we would propose for human memory is likely to be highly idiosyncratic. No one human can be expected to have a memory organization exactly like another. Indeed, what we call intelligence may be no more than reasonable versus unreasonable memory organization procedures (Schank, 1980).

On the other hand, all this does not mean that we cannot make a stab at differentiating among possible TOPs. The task is to find the right level of abstract description that is useful across domains. We are looking for the principles behind memory organization. TOPs that reflect those principles, although they might reorganize themselves, would still maintain their basic commonalities despite particular experiences.

Other TOP uses

One of the most important uses for TOPs is in conversation. Consider the following argument:

Israeli: Why don't the Arabs recognize the existence of Israel?
Arab: Why doesn't Israel conform to UN resolution 242?
Israeli: Because the resolution says that every state in the region must have the right to exist within secure and recognized borders, we would like to have secure borders first.
Arab: But what about the rights of the Palestinians to a secure homeland?

The above conversation is illustrative of another of the uses of TOPs. In conversations, we do more than simply answer questions that have been asked of us. We also think about what we have been asked. In doing so, we formulate an answer that puts forth our point of view. We make especially sure to do this when we are in an argument or an academic discussion. In order to put forth a point of view while not totally disregarding the question we have been asked, we must find relevant information in our memories that relates the topic of what we have been asked to our point of view on that subject.

If this is done in a very specific way, that is, if the topic of sentence 1 above is narrowly construed to be the recognition of Israel, then the requisite generality needed for the kind of answers we are discussing would be lost. TOPs are needed here so that specific inputs can be processed by general structures that contain memories that relate to those inputs in an interesting way. Formulating a good response to an assertion often requires one to draw analogies from other contexts.

We are not arguing here that TOPs contain the rules for generating a response. Rather, we are suggesting that the rules that a speaker does have need relevant memories to operate on. Further, we are suggesting that conversations of this sort depend heavily on a sort of *intentional reminding*. That is, an understander seeks, in his processing of a new input in a conversation, to be reminded of a memory that relates to what he heard and provides evidence for the point of view he wishes to defend.

In order for the Arab in the above argument to be able to respond to sentence 1 with 2, he must analyze 1 in the following way: First he must formulate an initial straightforward response to the input. Here this initial response is something like "Why should we do something for you?" To formulate this response, the Arab had to look up **Israel** in memory, find out that they were his enemy, look up **recognition,** find out what it is and that it is what Israel wants. At this point a TOP is easily found because the notion of **enemy** leads rather directly to that of a **competition goal.**

The next problem is to identify the conditions on the goal type that was found so that a TOP can be utilized. To do this, the Arab has many options available. He can look for solution conditions, result conditions and so on. These will be discussed at length in the next section. Let us assume that the Arab has decided to consider, as a possible avenue of thought about the subject of the question to him, the solution conditions for the problem. That is, he has in essence asked himself, "What can be done about a competition goal?" He knows that one possibility is compromise. He selects that path and thus finds the TOP: Competition Goal; Compromise Solution (CG;CS).

Notice that a TOP such as CG;CS is of great generality, but that it nevertheless pertains to this situation. Memories stored there will include prior known compromises, problems with compromises and so on. The understander thus has a wide range of memories available to him at this point. To come up with an actual response, he must provide his own indices.

In our prior examples of processing with TOPs, those indices were already provided. The problem there was for the understander to follow what had been said until he came to a relevant memory. The input itself informed the understander of what the TOPs and the indices in the TOPs were going to be.

Here, that is not the case. It is not in the Israeli's interest to provide the Arab with a good response, so he does not point to where a good one can be found. Nor does a good understanding of what the speaker has said require such a complex analysis. But a good response that is in the Arab's interest does require such effort.

Thus, TOPs are used here in a manner different from that discussed in the reminding examples. Because of this, a new problem for the understander is the selection of good indices. These indices should reflect both the situation described in the input and the intentions of the understander with respect to the formulation of a new response. In the example, one index would likely be the Middle East problem. This is not absolutely necessary however. It is certainly possible to go to a different level of conversation by discussing an analogous conflict in history that also happens to be stored in CG;CS.

The second index depends on the Arab's intentions. To formulate response 2 above, the index would have had to be *Arab's demands*. In indexing in a TOP, characteristics of that TOP are used in the index. Thus, in a CG;CS, the compromise that the Arab wanted would be a good index for him to use. Indexing in TOPs will be discussed in Chapter 11.

The memory about resolution 242 that is found in this way, together with the intention to assert the Arab's needs here (and some knowledge about how questions can be used in arguments), is sufficient to produce sentence 2.

The Israeli's response to 2 is more or less an answer to the question the Arab asked. It uses the same TOP, CG;CS, with the indices of *Israel's needs* and of *resolution 242*.

The Israeli response brings up the topic of secure borders. Here again CG;CS is necessary for understanding what the Israeli said and formulating the response. The indices this time are secure borders and again Arab needs. These indices cause the Palestinians' need for borders to be found in the Arab's memory.

Goals and conditions

We are now ready to consider more carefully what makes up a TOP. We have said that a TOP has both a goal type and a condition on that goal. The goal type must be one that involves the relationship of two parties with respect to the goal.

The first question to ask in our examination of possible goal types in TOPs is what aspects of goals are significant enough for us to organize memories around. To put this another way, what natural categories of goals are likely candidates for memory organization?

We will first make the following gross categorization. With respect to a given goal, we are likely to comment on, and thus to need to remember things about, the following aspects of any goal:

1. Problems during the pursuit of the goal.
2. Issues relating to what happens after a goal succeeds or fails. Within this gross division, there are the following goal types:

> PURSUIT
> mutual goal pursuit
> competition goals
> individual goal pursuit
>
> RESULTS
> achievement of success
> unanticipated side-effects
> goal blockage
> inconsistent goals

Within these basic goal types, there are sets of possible conditions. A condition is something that characterizes a particular aspect of the given goal type. Some conditions for the first two goal types are:

> MUTUAL GOAL PURSUIT
> outside opposition
> outside help
> difficulties along the way
> strange strategies
> apparent success
> apparent failure
>
> COMPETITION GOAL
> compromise solution
> opponent quits
> opponent gets stronger
> outside help
> difficulties along the way
> strange strategies
> apparent success
> apparent failure
> despicable tactics by opponent
> opponent changes colors

The above are illustrative of the kinds of TOPs that there are. Similar TOPs exist for the possibilities associated with success and failure. One of these we have already used is ACHIEVE SUCCESS; UTILIZE POWER in the Nixon and the Mayor of New Haven story.

More reminding

The primary issue with respect to TOPs is their usefulness as memory structures and hence as processing structures. While MOPs are specific to a given domain, TOPs encode domain-independent knowledge. TOPs contain information that will apply in many different domains. Clearly we have such domain-independent knowledge. The question is whether memories are stored in terms of such structures. Note here that we are not suggesting that any memory is stored only in terms of TOPs. As we suggested in Chapter 6, there are MOPs that contain knowledge pertinent to negotiations and treaties. But there are also TOPs active in such situations that are useful for bringing in memories involving other domains of knowledge that may have relevance in the current situation.

Thus, for example, CG;CS might well be an active TOP in a negotiation story.

Let us now consider two reminding experiences:

Case I

X was about to go out for lunch with Y. Y specifically asked X to go to a restaurant that served pizza because Y was on a diet and would be able to order one slice of pizza at this restaurant. X agreed. When they got there Y ordered two slices. This reminded X of the time that he went out to dinner with Z. X wanted to go to a Mexican restaurant and Z was on a diet so she wanted fish. She suggested a Mexican restaurant that served fish. X didn't like this restaurant but he agreed. When they got there Z ordered salad (which she could have gotten at any Mexican restaurant).

Case J

When W heard the above story she was reminded of making an appointment with a student at the only time the student could make it. This time was very inopportune for W but she agreed. At the agreed upon time, the student failed to show up.

Both of the above stories use the TOP we had used before for the argument that we mentioned above, namely COMPETING GOAL; COMPROMISE SOLUTION (CG;CS). The indices in case I are *diet, restaurant, feeling had,* and the characterization *reneged on promise.* In case J we have CG;CS and the *reneged on promise* and *feeling had* indices. Cases I and J and the Middle East Crisis share nothing in common in the way of context, yet they rely upon the same structure in memory for storage and learning. The consequence of this is not that one episode is likely to remind someone of the other (the indices would be different), but that information about how to deal with people in such situations can be applied across contexts.

Thus, various types of learning might take place. We might expect that next time X will be less likely to agree to a compromise with a person who is dieting when it comes to choosing restaurants. That is the lowest level conclusion possible here. Across contexts, if X were one of the Arab or

Israeli negotiators, it is possible he would be more skeptical of deals in those domains as well. It may not seem logical to apply what happened to you in a restaurant to a decision about an international negotiation, but people make such domain-crossing conclusions all the time. Sometimes such transferral across domains is exactly the right thing to do. Sometimes generalizations derived in this way are quite silly. Nevertheless, people can learn from experiences across contexts. That is, it is possible to draw a conclusion such as "never trust anybody under five feet three" from cases I and J as well. If X is the negotiator and his counterpart is under five foot three we might expect him to apply what he has learned. Whether he does or not, the point is that people have the ability to draw high level conclusions from what they experience. TOPs are required in order to get these remindings and in order to learn from these remindings.

Other types of TOPs

Consider case K:

Case K

X was talking about how there was no marijuana around for a month or two. Then, all of a sudden, everyone was able to get as much as they wanted. But the price had gone up 25 percent. This reminded X of the oil situation the previous year. We were made to wait on lines because of a shortage that cleared up as soon as the price had risen a significant amount.

The TOP that we propose as the one active in case K is POSSESSION GOAL: COMMODITY UNAVAILABLE (PG;CU). There are, of course, a great many possible plans available for possessing something. In Schank and Abelson (1977), we discussed the plan D-CONTROL, which contained seven planboxes for getting what you wanted. Some of these were ASK; BARGAIN; THREATEN; and OVERPOWER. Now we are suggesting that just as is the case with scripts, plans are also memory and processing structures at the same time. Thus, the particular methods we use can serve to organize memories, as do scripts. But, it seems clear that a structure such as POSSESSION GOAL; ASK is much too general. It is unlikely that such a structure would be useful since far too many experiences would be categorized under it.

(Let us emphasize again that no structure we propose is *right*. Any memory structure can be used until it contains too much or too little. Then it must be abandoned. Any dynamic self-organizing memory must have the ability to create and abandon structures as seen fit. We can only suggest here what the principles of such an organization might be.)

The organization we propose here is based again on the significant conditions that affect the planning for the possession goal. COMMODITY UNAVAILABLE alters the notion of the kind of planning that must be done. That is, knowing that a commodity is unavailable, we do not go through the litany of "Should I ask for it", "Should I bargain for it?", and so on. Rather, we plan according to the situation.

This particular story has only a peripheral relationship with planning, however. The planning knowledge is learned here. The next time a commodity becomes unavailable, we would expect X to think, "I'll just wait for a while. It will be available soon at a higher price." The lack of validity of this rule in a world different from the one in which X lives is irrelevant.

The indices in case K then are: *becomes available later, higher price,* and perhaps *controlled by unethical people.* We would also expect that the conclusion drawn from case K, (i.e., unethical people who control the commodity will put it back on the market when they've raised the price) would also serve as an index to the TOP PG;CU after case K had been processed.

We have previously seen an example of TOP similar in nature to PG;CU in the Afghanistan story. That TOP was POSSESSION GOAL; EVIL IN-TENT. In general, possession goals are an important part of TOPs. By extension, a great many other goal types can also form the basis of a TOP. Thus, we add to the list of TOPs given above, those TOPs that relate to the constraint involved in achieving a particular type of goal: Thus we have, for example:

> POSSESSION GOAL
> evil intent
> commodity unavailable
> dirty tactics
> commodity found unsatisfactory
>
> SATISFACTION GOAL
> object found doesn't satisfy
> novel solution
> choice between goal objects
> object chosen; second object better
>
> CRISIS GOAL
> normal solution doesn't work
> crisis abates mysteriously
> solution works for wrong reasons

A look at the TOPs shown here points out the obvious fact that more than one TOP can be active at a given time. We have knowledge about the situations that goals occur in as well as information specific to the pursuit of any particular goal. Thus, somebody can be in a goal competition situation for a possession goal. In that case TOPs of both types will carry expectations and memories that will be relevant. Because this is the case, it can be seen that the conditions in each TOP must be dependent upon the nature of the goal being characterized. That is, each condition must depend on whatever unique quality the goal part of the TOP contains. That uniqueness is what specifies its condition.

So far then, we have proposed a set of high level memory structures that relate to different aspects of what is going on in a situation. In general we want to be able to apply two kinds of memories to help us understand a new input at this level. First, we want to apply knowledge that has nothing to do with the particular goal we are tracking. Such information is about goals pursued in that situation in general, regardless of what actual goal it is. Second, we want to apply memories that are about the kind of goal we are tracking. Obviously we know some things about specific goal types that we would like to have available to us when necessary.

For example, the *Ostrich and the Sunbather* is possibly reached by two TOPs. Information about Ostriches can be categorized using a *hiding* index inside PRESERVATION GOAL; APPARENTLY SUCCESSFUL PLAN. On the other hand, it could be found, as would have had to have been the case here since the sunbather was not pursuing a preservation goal, by using GOAL BLOCKED;PLANNER UNAWARE.

It is important to understand that memories must be multiply-indexed in this fashion. (We say multiply because there are many other possibilities here. The ostrich information can be found with respect to our knowledge about ostriches, zoos, hiding and various MOPs that an ostrich might participate in, if any.) Multiple indexing is one source of our intelligence and of our ability to learn. This, of course, implies a multiple categorization of an input event, which, while difficult, is obviously a key issue in understanding.

A look at it all

What, then, have we said about TOPs? We have said that they are formed by goal types combined with conditions, often about planning, specific to those goal types. They are searched via indices that provide the specific trail to actual memories organized by the TOP.

Some TOPs employ general goal types. Their conditions relate to the goal type. Thus, conditions on goal-pursuit relate to the pursuit itself or to the result of the pursuit.

For other TOPs, the goal types are specific to a certain kind of goal.

Their conditions relate to the nature of that goal specifically. Thus, information about the success or failure of a possession goal belongs in the TOP for goal pursuit. Only information specifically related to the possession part of the possession goal belongs in the more specific TOP that encodes information about possession goals.

Part III

Generalization and learning

8   Generalization and memory

Developing and altering structures

There are two crucial issues that we can now address: the problem of the creation of new structures in memory, and that of the manipulation and alteration of already existing structures. The first of these problems has to do with the building of structures to deal with situations that are being encountered for the first time. The second has to do with new and unexplained information about previously understood aspects of the world.

People have widely differing experiences and must deal with equally differing sets of situations in the world. To keep track of these experiences and cope with these situations, each individual must create and maintain his own memory in processing structures. Clearly no one single set or configuration of structures could be used to explain the diversity of understanding and skills that we see in the world. It seems quite unlikely, then, that any particular structures are innate, though the ability to form and manipulate such structures may very well be.

No two people are likely to have identical structures except where those structures reflect the physical nature of the world or when those two people must function in identical societal arrangements. Even there, our experiences alter an individual's view of the world to such an extent that we can expect major differences. From a far enough distance away, any two members of the same physical or social world are likely to have similar mental structures. But viewed up close, these structures will contain distinct personal experiences.

As rigidly codified as behavior in a restaurant is, one person's experiences in a resaurant will not be the same as another's. This will lead people to different expectations. When expectations fail, they are the source of interesting generalizations, and this will happen to different people in different ways. Any individual will have his own peculiar expectations. Different expectations will fail to be fulfilled for different people.

Different generalizations will be made by different people. And, different experiences will serve to validate or invalidate those generalizations.

Thus, we can expect that people will have rather different MOPs, meta-MOPs, scenes, and scripts. The questions for us, then are: how do these structures get built in the first place; how do existing structures get altered once they have been built; and finally, how do new structures get created out of a reorganization of old structures?

In Chapter 6 we discussed briefly how one kind of memory, scripts, might come to exist in human memory. We hypothesized that the basic entity of human understanding is the *personal script,* the private expectations about how things proceed in one's life on a day to day or minute to minute basis.

In this chapter we will see how we begin to build up expectations about what other people will do in a variety of situations. Further, we will see how these expectations form the basis of our high level knowledge structures, and how these structures enable learning.

Building a personal script

The simple premise of personal script building is that anything that has happened in a certain way will happen that way again. To build a personal script, then, requires us to be able to do two things. First we must be able to recognize that a current experience is in some way similar to one that has occurred previously. Second, we must be able to focus on the important aspects of both episodes and eliminate from consideration those aspects of the current situation that are irrelevant to the retrieved memory. Recognizing that a situation is the same, in some significant ways, as the one we encountered previously and stored as a script is the key to our initial attempts at learning. This we call the *recognition problem.* (Others who have worried about this problem are Minsky, 1975; Charniak, 1977; and DeJong, 1979.) The problem of centering our attention on the relevant aspects of the similarity between two episodes is called the *focus problem.*

A major issue with respect to the recognition problem, is establishing the kinds of structures that must be recognized. By defining such structures generally enough, the number of structures that must be recognized is more limited. Given that we have proposed the scene as a basic structure in memory, we must concern ourselves with how scenes are defined, and how scenes are established initially, i.e., how can we address the recognition problem for scenes?

We have argued that the features that determine a scene are varied.

While they include physical information of the sort available to a child, they also include goals, intentions, and social dynamics that are likely to be unknown to him. Thus, at the simplest level, a scene is physically determined. When a child learns to identify certain patterns of actions that recur as personal scripts, then he does so in terms of the physical scene that surrounds those actions. As we will see however, this physical awareness alone will be inadequate for the processing of much of what a child experiences.

At the same time that a child is building a script, he is also beginning to build MOPs. If a scene is physically bounded, and a script is limited by that boundary, then any other actions that regularly co-occur with a scene, but occur in a different physical location, must be stored in terms of a different, but connected scene. Connecting scenes together is the role of MOPs. Thus, at the same time that a child begins to develop personal scripts, he must also be developing scenes and MOPs. These three kinds of high level knowledge structures are developed in parallel.

Expectations are primarily scene-connected in the small child. But what typifies a scene for a child of about six months of age? Children of that age appear to have some notion of a script. A small child has only a small number of different physical locations that he is likely to be in. But a scene is made up of more than just physical location. Being in the crib and crying is probably a different scene for a child from being in the crib and playing with a toy. Or, to put this another way, a child is likely to have expectations about the first situation that do not apply in the latter. A scene is a combination of physical aspects and goals. A child's notion of an adult's goals may not be very sophisticated. In fact, a child probably has no idea why his parents do what they do. Still, a child has his own goals and expectations of how his parents will react to what he does to achieve them.

Thus, we might expect a six-month-old child to have something like the following scenes (with related goals):

> TABLE-SITTING (and hungry)
> CRIB (and desire to not be wet)
> CRIB and JUST WOKE UP
> PLAYPEN (and crying for lack of attention)
> STROLLER and BEING-PUSHED-ON-THE-SIDEWALK
> STROLLER and STORE
> CAR
> HIGH-CHAIR and RESTAURANT

A script is primarily a set of expectations about what will happen in a given situation. In particular, we would expect that attached to each of these scenes would be the child's expectations about what his parent is likely to do when the scene is activated. In other words, the child has at least one personal script attached to each of the above scenes.

Three questions remain:

> How does the child develop those personal scripts?
> How does the child create MOPs from the scripts?
> How does the child alter the structures he has created?

Continuing on with the assumption that there are three kinds of MOPs, we believe that it is likely that each of the MOP types is organized to its base around a common element that derives initially from what one can perceive at an early age. Before we explain how this happens, it is important to consider what it means to organize a scene *at its base*.

When a child has three or four things that he has perceived about his environment that he considers to be important (and certainly this is an oversimplification), in order to be able to store those three or four items as one unit (a scene) to be recognizable later, he must elect one of those items as primary. This is the *first discrimination* in a discrimination net scheme. Whatever indexing method is used, one aspect of the situation must be noticed first, and a second aspect must be *looked for* (indexed) in terms of the first. From a process point of view, in a set of ordered steps, something must come first.

This decision, that certain things are primary and others secondary, seems uncomfortably arbitrary. But, in growing structures, such decisions must be made. This is part of what was referred to as the *focus problem* above. One way around this problem is to make use of the difference between the three types of MOPs – physical, societal, and personal. That is, given three major aspects of the situation, each one representative of one of the types of MOPs, no selection is necessary. Rather, three parallel structures are created, each with a different one of the items at the base. In other words, the child finds himself not in one scene, but in three different scenes. All three scenes need not exist simultaneously in the child's head. It is certainly possible that a child will choose to follow one of them and ignore the others. The point is mainly that the potential exists for three scenes.

Now let us consider what these three scenes are. From the point of view of a baby, the three MOP types translate into:

> Physical: the features of the world around him
> Societal: what other people are around
> Personal: what feelings and sensations does he feel

A scene can be developed around any of these three aspects of a situation. Once a scene is decided upon, the series of events that take place next are encoded as a set of expectations attached to that scene. However, unless a scene is sensibly defined in the first place, deciding where events begin and end in a script attached to a scene can be difficult. For example, after a baby has his diaper changed he may be carried off to another room. Such a physical change would destroy one of the major aspects of the scene and thus help to close off any diaper-changing script that the child was learning. But, suppose this child were played with in his crib after diaper changing. How does the child know if that should be part of *$DIAPER-CHANGE* or not? As it turns out this is a serious problem for parents and babies. A child who experiences A followed by B will continue to expect B every time he experiences A, even after many failures of that expectation. (When I was six, my mother baked cookies and put them in the ice bucket. Every time after that, when the ice bucket was put out in anticipation of a party, I hopefully opened it. Never again were cookies stored there, but the hopeful expectation remained for many years.)

The problem of growing a personal script, requires the ability to make guesses and later correct them. (Note that this is not done in order to create a script. Rather, it is done in order to understand.) In rough outline, the process looks like this:

Perceive aspects of scene
For each scene aspect:

1. Observe actions
2. Create expectation that those actions will repeat the next time the scene is encountered
3. Modify expectations whenever they are violated
4. Alter existing script by changing failure-indexed expectations
5. Elevate repeated expectation failures to the status of new scripts

Building a personal script then, requires us to take a set of actions and states and associate them with a scene. The next time that scene is encountered, the prior actions and states are expected.

When the new input actions fail to correspond to the set of actions or states that obtained last time, there are the following possibilities:

A. Modify specific expectation
B. Alter script itself
C. Index as expectation failure

We will now consider each of these in turn.

Dealing with expectation failure

The dominating notion in building and altering memory structures is expectation-failure. In order to discover what the options are when an

expectation fails, consider some examples that might well occur in the life
of a small child:

A. *Expectation Modification*
When a child has eaten only hamburgers in restaurants, we can presume that he
would have an expectation that he gets hamburgers when he eats in a restaurant. Upon having a hot dog ordered, he will have to modify his script expectation. This corresponds to what we shall call *learning the variables*. That is, the
child must learn what parts of his expectations are firm and what parts must be
given enough flexibility to withstand changes. Ideally, the child does not want to
have to create a completely new expectation for ordering, eating and so on,
based upon this discrepancy.

B. *Script Alteration*
In an adult, scripts at the level we have been talking about are scene-specific and
rather rigid. Thus, there is really very little variability in them. They correspond
roughly in form to what we called an *instrumental script* in Schank and Abelson
(1977). The child's task therefore, in his quest to supply himself with a set of adult
scripts, is to attempt to separate out the invariant elements in what he observes
and place them in one unit as a mental structure.

C. *Indexing Expectation Failures*
Now we get to the heart of the matter. Scripts must be organized in such a way
that they carry information particular to the circumstances they describe. At the
same time, we want general information to be available to help. In the circumstances we described above, we want an ordering script to contain restaurant-
specific information. At the same time we want the ORDER scene to contain
information about ordering in general that will be available for use at appropriate
parts of the $ORDER script. How can this all be configured?

Returning to our child in the crib with a wet diaper, let us imagine
that this child is always played with after his diaper is changed. Let us
further assume that this play takes place in the crib. There is no particular reason that the child should realize that **diaper changing** and **playing
in the crib** are unrelated. In fact, in his world they are most certainly
related. But, the child will eventually experience diaper changing in a
different environment. Further, he will experience **playing in the crib**
without diaper changing. We would like our child to be able to apply
what he has learned from a diaper change outside the crib to one inside
the crib. Similarly, if he has learned a game in the crib, we would like
him to be able to ask for it in another circumstance. To do this, he must
separate these two events from each other. This is what we call MOP
creation.

MOP creation takes place every time two scenes are seen to function
independently from one another while also frequently occurring in sequence. The expectation that they will occur in tandem in some circumstances is not lost despite their newly discovered independence. This
expectation is maintained by creating a structure in memory that records

the relationship between the other two structures, i.e., a MOP. In this case we would have a MOP called M-CRIB SEQUENCE consisting of two scenes: CRIB-WET and CRIB-PLAY. Each of these scenes has its appropriate script attached.

A somewhat more realistic example can be found in restaurants. A child may go in the car only to travel to restaurants, and he may always go to restaurants in a car. Nevertheless CAR and RESTAURANT should become two quite different and unrelated structures for an adult. CAR is a scene that may have a number of scripts related to it. RESTAURANT is a MOP that consists of many different scenes (such as ORDER, EAT) connected to each other in a variety of ways. The child, in noting the independence of these entities, must create a structure to connect them. But as M-RESTAURANT is a MOP, what he must construct is something that can take M-RESTAURANT as one of its pieces. (In this case something like mM-TRIP applies, although the child could not construct such an entity at this point.) The problem here in *meta-MOP creation* is to also be able to make the scene CAR into a variable in a larger structure so that it is seen as one of many modes of possible transportation to a place that you wish to go to do something, and so that M-RESTAURANT is seen as one of many possible things to do. This process is quite complex.

At the risk of overstating the point, let us diverge a moment to discuss M-RESTAURANT. Note that it follows from what we have been saying about creating MOPs and making place holders in MOPs that will take scenes as variables that ORDER, EAT and so on must become structures in their own right. That is, we can separate out EAT from the restaurant experience and discover that what we learn in that situation applies when we are not in a restaurant. Certainly, if you discover that a certain kind of fish disagrees with you, even though recalling that should bring to mind the restaurant scene in which that discovery took place, it would be foolish to suggest that the actor in this event would fail to remember this experience when eating in someone's home. Similar arguments obtain between something learned when ordering in a restaurant that might apply when ordering in a store. Knowledge relevant to persuading the clerk to get you what you want might well come from some restaurant experience. This is why RESTAURANT must be a MOP and not a script. The scripts here are *$RESTAURANT-ORDER, $RESTAURANT-PAY,* and so on. But these scripts are attached to scenes that are more general (ORDER and PAY) that include knowledge available from other settings.

We argued earlier that when an expectation generated by a script fails, an index is created at that point, to the memory of the experience that caused the failure. The index, we argued, was either an explanation of the failure itself or a significant aspect of the failure experience. Now consider a four year old child in a restaurant. Viewed as a physical entity only, restaurant ordering looks only like restaurant ordering. Therefore the set of expectations built up by his ordering in a restaurant would be restaurant-specific. Now, let us imagine that one of these expectations fails. For example, suppose the child says "Get me the ketchup." and the waitress gets mad and leaves. We want the child to mark this failure in his ordering script and attempt to explain it.

Now consider a different expectation failure. In this hypothetical example, the child orders a hamburger and it comes back burnt. This is also an expectation failure, but it is a failure of a different kind. In the first case, the child failed to get what he wanted. This is true in the second case as well. But the explanations are radically different in the two cases. In particular, the explanations differ in their implications for how behavior must be modified in the future. It is future behavior modification that is the essence of the problem. In other words, if the child learns effectively from both of these situations, we would expect that he would be more polite as a result of the first failure and, in response to the second, perhaps he would ask his parents not to go to that restaurant again, or not to order hamburgers again.

Where will this new knowledge reside? In the first case, the knowledge of how to talk politely to waitresses could readily be incorporated into *$RESTAURANT-ORDER*. But if it did, the child would not be able to apply what he had learned from this experience to ordering in other situations. Clearly, this is the kind of expectation failure than results in modifying the scene ORDER rather that the particular script in ORDER. ORDER is part of the MOP M-RESTAURANT, which is a physical MOP. The script *$RESTAURANT-ORDER* is indexed under ORDER and is responsible for detailing the physical behavior of the waitress and the customer (coming to the table, reading the menu, etc.) For an adult, ORDER also fills a place holder in M-CONTRACT (which has been implicity activated by M-RESTAURANT) for specifying the details of the negotiation for delivery. The failure should be marked in ORDER, rather than in the MOPs or scripts that relate to ORDER.

Thus, higher level learning and generalization take place by indexing a given expectation failure in terms of the MOPs, scenes, and scripts that were active whenever the expectation failure occurred. Not all expectation failures have such global ramifications. We shall now consider this issue in more detail.

Expectation failures and the modification of structures

The first problem we must face here is assessing what kinds of expectation failures there are and how each affects the various structures that are likely to be active at the time that an expectation was generated. That is, we must consider how expectation failures alter active memory structures.

From that perspective, a failed expectation can do any of the following:

1. Modify the expectations in the script from which it was generated
2. Modify the scene that the script was called from
3. Modify the MOP that the scene was called from
4. Modify the meta-MOP that the MOP was called from
5. Cause a new script to be generated
6. Cause a new scene to be generated
7. Cause a new MOP to be generated
8. Cause a new meta-MOP to be generated

In other words, an expectation failure can modify the variables in an expectation, create a new expectation, or delete an old expectation within an existing structure.

Thus, there are two issues:

How do we know which structure should be modified by an expectation failure?
How do we know whether to modify an existing structure or create a new one?

The problem is to be able to analyze why an expectation has failed. We do not modify our existing knowledge structures until we have some new knowledge to add to them. New knowledge does not come automatically because an expectation fails. The new knowledge we are seeking comes from attempting to explain an expectation failure. The real issue here is finding an algorithm for creating explanations of unexpected events.

Explaining expectation failure

Let us consider some of the expectaion failures that we have seen in previous chapters to illustrate some of the possibilities that exist for alteration of existing structures and the creation of new ones.

When an expectation generated by an existing knowledge structure fails, its failure is marked with a pointer from the expectation to the memory that exemplifies the failure of that expectation. The pointer optimally carries with it an explanation of the failure, so that the system can know under what circumstances it should use this information.

To make this more concrete, consider the Legal Seafood case from Chapter 2. After processing an episode at Legal Seafood, we would want to have detected a MOP-based expectation failure and have so indexed it.

Why is this a MOP-based failure and how does a system know what structure to alter? The MOP M-RESTAURANT indicates the order of occurrence of scenes in a sequence. One way, then, that a MOP can fail is by having the ordering of scenes that it predicts turn out to be wrong. In Legal Seafood, the PAYING scene comes immediately after the ordering scene. Thus M-RESTAURANT would be marked, at least initially, with an index after ORDER that PAY came next in this particular instance. But, simply marking M-RESTAURANT is not enough.

The main question that is generated by any expectation failure is: What alteration of the structure responsible for that expectation must be made? In general, we can look at this as a two-step problem. First we must identify the conditions that obtained when the failure occurred. Once this is done we must decide whether the failure in quetion is indicative of a failure in the knowledge structure itself, or just of a specific expectation in that structure. The first part of this involves the determination of how a current context differs from situations in which the failed expectation was valid. The second involves the determination of what aspect of a structure should be altered to accommodate the current failure.

This final alteration of structure takes three forms: alteration of a specific expectation within the structure; abandonment and replacement of the entire structure; or reorganization of the placement of the structure. In terms of our restaurant example these three possibilities work out to be:

1. M-RESTAURANT could be altered by attaching to one of its expectations a pointer to an episode where that expectation failed.
2. M-RESTAURANT could be abandoned as a failed MOP. One or more new MOPs would then be constructed to replace it.
3. M-RESTAURANT would be unaltered except in terms of the conditions under which it was called up in the first place. Those conditions would be altered to point to a new MOP under the conditions that obtained in the episode that caused the failure and to M-RESTAURANT otherwise.

These three possibilities – alteration, replacement, and reorganization – are, in general, possibilities that occur any time an expectation fails. How do we choose from among them?

In the case of a failure that does not produce a reminding, that is a failure that is happening for the first time, the choice is clear. We take the event that surrounds the failure and, once having decided what expectation is responsible for the failure, index the failure under the expectation to blame. This is what reminding is about. Reminding, in one of its most common forms, illustrates the use of the storage of an episode in terms of a failed expectation. That storage was made as a way of holding off the decision on whether to alter existing MOPs pending further experiences of the same sort.

In the cases in which the failure does in fact cause us to be reminded of a similar failure in the past we are faced with the need to create a new structure to handle what are now seen not as failures, but as repeated and possibly normal aspects of a situation. This new structure will itself have expectations that anticipate the events which were once seen as failures. The question in this case, then, is whether to replace the old structure altogether, or to simply reorganize memory to accommodate the use of both the old and new structures.

The answer to this question depends upon the confidence associated with the original structure, and confidence depends, for the most part, upon frequency of use. In cases where the old structure has never been used without the incidence of failure, or has never been used at all, we would tend to replace. In the case of a frequently used structure, however, we would reorganize our memory to incorporate both the old and new structures, along with a means to get to the correct one at the correct time.

Now we can consider our visitor to Burger King and McDonald's. A first encounter with Burger King, for a person whose knowledge structures contain only the standard M-RESTAURANT, would produce an expectation failure in the order of

ORDER, SEATING, PAY.

When multiple failures occur, it is a good bet that it is because the MOP being used was of little value. Thus, in a situation of multiple failure, a new MOP must be constructed. This construction is complex since it involves reworking the existing MOP to create the new one. This is done by altering the MOP first, and the scenes second, as follows.

As in the Legal Seafood example, in Burger King PAY goes right after ORDER. In fact, we might expect a reminding here if Legal Seafood were experienced first. We have an additional problem with respect to M-RESTAURANT in that the SEATING scene follows PAY and ORDER. Further there are some script expectation failures, too. For example, $RESTAURANT-ORDER is not usually done while standing.

The first thing that must be done then is construct a new MOP. Assuming that M-RESTAURANT has a high confidence attached to it in our hypothetical memory, we decide to reorganize rather than replace. (It is certainly plausible that this assumption is not actually the case. For many children, Burger King might in fact be the basis of what they know about restaurants.)

To construct a new MOP, we start with the scenes of the old MOP and reorder them according to the new episode. This is easy in the case of what we will temporarily call M-BURGER KING. But, while the scenes may be the same, the scripts are different. A scene describes what takes place in general. And, in general, what takes place in a regular restaurant and a fast-food restaurant is the same. But the specifics are different. We do not want to use the scripts associated with M-RESTAURANT, therefore. We want to construct new scripts. Actually, since the new script is identical to the first Burger King episode, the real problem is to alter the scenes.

At this point we have a new MOP, M-BURGER KING, that contains the scenes ENTER + ORDER + PAY + SEATING with very specific scripts attached to each scene. Two problems remain. First we must encode the scripts correctly in the scene. Second we must make M-BURGER KING more abstract so that it is a MOP that is more likely to be of great use, namely M-FAST FOOD. These two problems are related.

The scene alteration problem depends, after all, on how a scene is constructed in the first place. Let us then, by way of example, consider the ORDER scene.

ORDER, as we have said, is a scene that is used by a great many MOPs. Some of these might include: M-RESTAURANT, M-SHOPPING, M-PRO-VIDE-SERVICE, M-OFFICE, M-TELEPHONE-BUYING, M-TRAVEL-AGENT. The scene ORDER, in order to be used by this diverse set of MOPs, must be written in as general a way as possible. ORDER is one of those scenes that is both physical and societal. That is, it expresses both the generalizations that are valid when someone is physically ordering something, and those that pertain to the relationship between the participants in an ORDERing situation. Below, we have the physical scene ORDER. It looks a lot like a script, but without any particulars. Particular scripts, pointed to by ORDER (for example, *$BURGER-KING ORDER, $FANCY RESTAURANT ORDER, $SUPPLY-ROOM ORDER*), fill in the details or *color* the ORDER scene. Here then, is one possible view of ORDER:

Participants: actor, agent
Props: desired object or service; medium of MTRANSing
Preconditions: actor can MTRANS to agent
   agent can be assumed to have ability to get object or do service
   agent has willingness to get object or do service
Actions: actor establishes MTRANS linkage
   actor questions possibility of service being performed or object being
   delivered
   actor questions price of object or service
   actor states desire to agent

agent agrees to comply
agent tells actor when compliance will be complete

Now, at first glance, such a scene may seem much too general. And, in fact, the above scene would probably not actually be used as is in any given situation. But it doesn't have to be. The role of a script attached to a scene is to color the scene with the particulars of that scene. In other words, a script is a copy of a scene with particulars filled in. For a script to be used, a copy of the scene is made that alters the scene in appropriate ways, leaving intact the parts of the scene that fit perfectly.

Here is the advantage of this scheme: Knowledge that is acquired from restaurants about ordering that applies to all kinds of ordering will be known to so apply because the piece that was acquired will have been copied unchanged from the scene. The only way such knowledge can apply across the board to all ordering is if it relates to a non-restaurant specific portion of the script. In other words, expectation failures that are script-specific are stored in terms of the script itself. But expectation failures that were due to expectations that were derived unchanged from a scene are stored in terms of the original scene.

To see how the scene-script relationship looks in practice, let us consider the script *$RESTAURANT-ORDER*. A script augments the scene that called it up by coloring it according to specific knowledge acquired about that script. When *$RESTAURANT-ORDER* colors ORDER it takes each line in it and either copies it directly or alters it to suit the script. For example, the precondition

agent has willingness to get object or do service

is a line in ORDER. *$RESTAURANT-ORDER* colors this line by adding the information that a waitress, because it is her job, can be assumed to have agreed to participate in the scene. Similarly the actions: actor questions possibility of service being performed or object being delivered and actor questions price of object or service are taken care of by the definition of a restaurant in the first case, and by a menu in the second. That is, *$RESTAURANT-ORDER* colors ORDER by replacing an abstract line about price with information about reading a menu. Thus, these lines are altered in this script to reflect known information about restaurants. In addition, a patron of a restaurant may have a great deal of specific knowledge about what is good to order. This would be found in a subscript indexed off the above script to be called up when appropriate.

Let us take a look at how a problem in ORDER can cause memory to be changed. Suppose we have a person who orders in a restaurant and

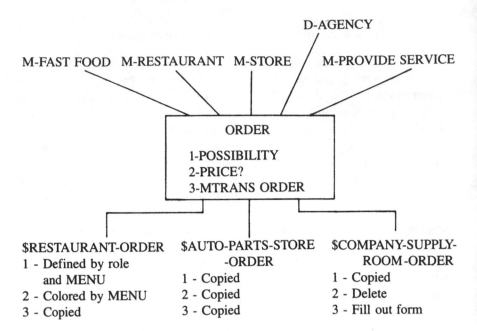

Figure 3

finds that he isn't served because he was nasty. Initially, this person might have a memory structure that looks like Figure 3.

This figure shows how the scene ORDER is used by three scripts. Those scripts have copied the information in ORDER and either replaced it by coloring, or copied it directly. Three MOPs that use ORDER as one of its scenes are also shown. In addition, the generalization of the goal behind ORDER, namely D-AGENCY, is also connected to ORDER. This relationship is close to a hierarchical superset relationship. The MOP connection is one of filler to empty slot.

Now let's consider what happens when this person's nasty order goes unfilled in the restaurant. First, there is an expectation failure. The episode is indexed off of *$RESTAURANT-ORDER* in slot 3. But, as slot 3 has been copied directly from the ORDER scene, this index is moved up to that level. When the same failure occurs in an auto parts store, or a fast food restaurant, or any other script that copies slot 3 directly from ORDER, a reminding occurs. This second instance causes a re-evaluation of the expectation that has failed. This re-evaluation causes an attempt to explain the failure.

In this case, the explanation is that servers like to be talked to politely.

Finding such explanations is an extremely complex process. Often they are not easily discoverable. We may need to be told; we may never find out. But when we do find an explanation, it enables us to modify ORDER in slot 3 accordingly. This allows every MOP that uses ORDER to have that fix incorporated in it without doing a thing. The new, altered, ORDER is simply used by any MOP that previously used the old ORDER. In other words, this hypothetical person should now remember to talk politely to anyone who is in a serving role.

In additon to this modification of ORDER, D-AGENCY is also modified. This is done because of the superset relationship that holds. The modification of any ASK in D-AGENCY (ORDER is connected as a method attached to ASK) has ramifications for all acenes that employ an ASK. Thus $RESTAURANT-ENTER, which also can use ASK (for a table), can be modified by this experience. Though the link to D-AGENCY is reached through ORDER then, this modification itself is not linked to M-RESTAURANT or ORDER in any way.

Note that if memory were not set up in the way we have suggested, that is, if $RESTAURANT-ORDER were connected directly to M-RESTAURANT, and $AUTO-PARTS-ORDER were connected directly to M-STORE, then failures would not be generalized optimally. That is, unless ORDER is affected no general learning would take place. If only the scripts, which have only a very local scoping, are affected, the scenes, which are used throughout the memory, would not be able to carry the knowledge learned from one context to another.

Now let us consider the Burger King example again. The problem in constructing M-BURGER KING is to take each scene that that MOP uses and treat each action that occurs within it in terms of its deviation from the baseline scene. Thus, $BURGER-KING-ORDER is built by noting how the actions observed in the first experience with Burger King differ from the ORDER scene.

The next step is, of course, that we want to change M-BURGER-KING into the more general M-FAST FOOD. To do this, it is necessary to index M-BURGER KING in terms of M-RESTAURANT. The reason for this is that we want a patron entering McDonald's for the first time to be reminded of Burger King. In other words, we want the patron to know to use M-BURGER-KING rather than M-RESTAURANT, and develop the specific M-BURGER-KING into the more useful M-FAST-FOOD by generalizing the roles and circumstances in which it can be called. How can this be accomplished? One way is to index M-BURGER-KING in M-RESTAURANT at the point of its failed expectation relevant to Burger King. In this case this would mean noting that the scene ordering was different in a particular way. A marker, then, would have to be placed in M-RESTAU-RANT at the point of the past expectation failure. This marker would itself direct the attention of the processor to both the episode in which the failure occurred, and M-BURGER-KING itself.

After this rerouting of processing has occurred a few times in the same way, the reminding ceases to occur. At that point M-BURGER-KING has been transformed into a MOP with entry conditions of its own, that is, one that can be called in for use without even seeing it as a deviant type of restaurant. To put this more generally, a new MOP is grown at the point where its conditions for use have been detected so that it can be called up independently from the MOP in which it originated as an expectation failure. Thus, after a few trials, M-RESTAURANT and M-FAST FOOD are independent MOPS.

Summary

When an expectation fails, it is necessary to trace the source of the expectation. Script-generated expectations cause modification of scripts by marking these failures. Repeated failures of the same kind cause new scripts or new MOPs to be generated. New scripts are generated when there is only one MOP controlling the flow of events and its expectations are confirmed. When more than one MOP is active, a variety of strategies are used for discovering what structure to modify.

When an expectation failure is MOP related, again one expectation failure can be marked as an index to memory, but two is cause for rethinking one's MOPs. (Or, a new MOP may be generated in response to one failure. It may never be generated at all for some people, no matter how many failures they experience.) Usually, new NOPs are generated as more experiences accrue in a given area, lending finer detail to one's knowledge of a situation.

The last expectation failure in our list is the scene-based expectation failure. This occurs when the script piece that generated the failed expectation turns out to have been copied directly from the scene. Such a failure can serve to begin a radical reorganization. To discuss it requires a careful discussion of scenes first. We shall deal with all this in the next chapter.

It could be argued from our previous discussions that the scene is the most
significant structure in memory. MOPs organize scenes. Scenes hold what is
general about scripts, and thus serve to organize scripts. In the middle
then, are scenes, holding actual memories and pointing to other scenes that
hold memories, and scripts (where expectation violations hold memories.)
It is imperative then, that we carefully define and discuss scenes.

But, as we said in the last chapter, a scheme where scripts are only
associated with a given physical scene will fail to capture enough generality. In order to learn effectively, it is necessary for a child to disembody
the scripts he has learned from the scenes they originally occurred in. He
must begin to see *$DIAPER CHANGE* as an entity by itself. But, should he
lose the connection between *$ DIAPER CHANGE* and CRIB? There would
seem no reason to do so. What he must do, however, is to associate
$DIAPER CHANGE with scenes such as PARENTAL INTERACTION and
PERSONAL COMFORT. That is, he must begin to store and understand
scripts in terms of scenes that are societal and personal rather than just
wholly physical. In this way societal and personal scenes come to domi-
nate scripts of their own in the child's memory.

This is all part of the evolution in the development of memory structures from the primacy of physical scenes to the three part division of
scenes that we have suggested. Additionally, there is a second development in memory structures taking place, namely the one from physically-
motivated physical scenes to goal-motivated physical scenes. Both of
these changes can be better examined by considering our old friend, the
restaurant.

From physical to societal

Initially, a restaurant is primarily defined by its physical characteristics.
We assume that a child sees a restaurant as a place that is large, noisy,

143

and so on, where you sit down and eat. In other words, a scene is initially defined by its primary physical characteristics and the overall intentions of the participants in the scene. The physical scene RESTAURANT does not cease to exist in the child's head as he grows older. Nevertheless, a set of societal and personal scenes evolves from that basic physical scene.

Consider ORDER again. The physical sight of the waitress coming to the table, standing by the table and writing on a pad, talking to people at the table and so on, is just as physically real as a restaurant. But, the weight of the participant's intentions is stronger in such a scene. As the child begins to see this as *ordering* rather than merely as *someone talking to you in a restaurant,* he must, if he is to learn from what he experiences, store information about this ordering in the ORDER scene. But, as this evolution takes place, the physical aspects of the scene do not go away. Rather, they also evolve into discrete pieces that set the background for events.

As we said in Chapter 6, there usually are at least three different MOPs active during any experience. These three MOPs, one for each type of scene, often will be calling upon three different scenes at the same time. At other times they will all be coloring the same scene. Thus, a child will eventually realize that M-CONTRACT, along with M-RESTAURANT, is helping to specify and explain the actions of the waitress. That is, he begins to see that what was once purely a physical issue for him has societal implications. He understands that M-RESTAURANT calls upon M-CONTRACT and that therefore it is possible to generalize from what happens in a restaurant to similar actions that happen in other places. That is, he can begin to see that there is some unity to what happens around him, and that often this unity is provided by societal roles. Thus, he can begin to generalize, and hence to learn from these identities.

Two people can witness the same events, yet remember them differently. An individual who has societal MOPs available to help interpret people's actions will be able to understand better than someone who has only physical MOPs to help. An example of this is witnessing (or reading about) an act of terrorism. Such an act can be seen purely physically (as a kidnapping for example), or it can be seen as a societal action. Thus, M-TERRORISM is similar to M-CONTRACT in that, despite whatever physical manifestation it might have, it can be seen as an instance of a negotiated agreement (in this case under threatening circumstances) between people.

> M-TERRORISM: [violent physical ACT] + DEMANDS + NEGOTIA-
> TIONS + AGREE + [physical ACT]

None of the scenes shown above are physical (except the place holders), nor can their physical means be directly inferred. Once we know that we have an embassy takeover, for example, we can use the correct MOP to fill in the physical ACT. M-EMBASSY TAKEOVER is a physical MOP. But, it is also an instantiation of M-TERRORISM. Both MOPs are active, each contributing something to the understanding of the situation. Because of this, an embassy takeover could be confused with a kidnapping, despite the fact that their physical realizations might be very different. The societal MOPs in each case are the same. Seeing actions that are different physically as identical societally, can enable learning since information garnered from one domain can be applied in another.

From physical to goal-based physical

Now let us return to our child in his crib. Here, we want the generalization that a crib, and its surrounding room, is best seen as an instance of a bedroom. Clearly, this can only be done if a transformation is made from a strictly physical interpretation of events in the room to one that includes the goal of those events. It is hard to say at what point a child learns to understand why people do what they do, but is is safe to say that he does do this at some point. So, for example, a bedroom has as it intention satisfying the goal of S-REST (see Schank and Abelson, 1977 for a discussion of such goals). At the point where the child realizes that his room also has this intentional aspect to it, and that it furthermore shares that intention with other rooms in the world, he can begin to *see* physical scenes in goal-based terms. The ability to see things this way is the start of the second evolution we were talking about, from purely physical scenes to goal-based physical scenes.

Scene-based expectation failures

We are now ready to answer the question of how an expectation failure causes us to modify a scene. We have seen that physical scenes are constantly evolving in two ways, first by taking on a societal aspect (modification due to other people's goals) and second by taking on a goal-based aspect (modification due to our own goals).

Consider the failure from ORDER that we discussed earlier. The child asks the waitress for ketchup, but does so obnoxiously, and thus does not get it. The expectation that the person whose role it is to serve will, when asked, serve, comes from ORDER. When this expectation fails, it is marked as a modification of ORDER to be consulted next time. This is done because it was ORDER's uncolored expectation, free from the script $RESTAURANT-ORDER, that failed. (Of course, the expectation might have been colored. For example, there might be a script, $DELICATESSEN-ORDER, where the rules for ordering are slightly different. Subtle distinctions of that kind are held in scripts, i.e., as colored expectations from scenes.)

We saw an example of the modification of ORDER before when we discussed ORDER as it relates to M-PROVIDE-SERVICE in the Steak and the Haircut example. In that example, asking for hair to be cut in a certain way is done under the auspices of the ORDER scene. The expectation failure that occurs when the haircut is not short enough is marked in ORDER by an index. This index is, in this case, an explanation of why the expectation failed. Here, the expectation failed because, according to Y in the story, the extreme degree of the request was not insisted upon. Thus, a new addition to ORDER is made by marking, at the point of *asking* in ORDER, that if extremeness is required it must be emphasized. The explanation for this new rule in ORDER is tied, by a pointer, to the Haircut experience. This explanation by example will effect remindings until the reminding has occurred sufficiently often to cause the new addition to become a standard part of the ORDER scene.

Now consider the child in the crib who has the expectation that he will be played with when his diaper is being changed. Suppose he is not played with. In that case the expectation that has failed comes from the scene. To fix this, the child must (unconsciously of course) figure out whether this failure is physical (that is, something that was part of his expectations about the physical scene) or societal (that is, something that was his expectation about what people in his life do with him). To us it is clearly the latter. (A child will find this distinction extremely troublesome, of course. Children are not one-shot learners.)

An important step of learning then, is the extraction of the personal events in a failed expectation. When an expectation fails, we must find out whether the reason it failed was in some sense idiosyncratic, or whether there is something about one's view of the world that was wrong. Expectation failures that depend upon personal attributes as opposed to societal or physical attributes, must be taken out of their original physical scene and treated separately. If they recur in another location, the hypothesis is confirmed, and a new personal scene is born. A problem of some importance for an understander then, is correctly identifying the nature of an expectation failure in order to determine if a new scene or MOP should be created as a result of that failure.

Personal scenes that are created as the explanation for expectation failures when societal or physical explanations would have been more appropriate, can be the basis for all sorts of psychological problems later on. Since, as we have argued, memory works in such a way as to group like experiences under a common heading, *parents failing your expectations by not playing with you during diaper changing* can become such a heading (or MOP) rather easily. The question is how often such newly created expectations get satisfied and how they get generalized. Frequent experiences of the same kind will solidify a MOP; in this case they will confirm one's fears about parental behavior. The issue is not how one's parents react in this one situation, of course. After some time, *diaper changing* stops. But expectations about *parents,* and generalizing from there, *loved ones,* and from there to *people,* continue to occur. Psychologically troubled people are likely to have negative sets of expectations (MOPs) about different people's behavior toward them, that will have been confirmed by their experience. These are personal MOPs and thus separate from *standard experience.*

A scene-based expectation that fails because its goal is satisfied without the scene being invoked is a more complex, and more significant kind of failure than the simpler expectation failure mentioned above. Consider the child who is put to bed for the first time in a strange room. The child has suffered an expectation failure of a goal-connected scene. That is, assuming that early on the goal of S-REST is connected with being in the CRIB scene, we can assume that attempting to satisfy S-REST in another scene will be distressing for a child. This distress is solved by a scene reorganization (although often parents anxious to quiet baby do not have the patience to wait the days or weeks that it might take for the child to realize that it is normal for sleep to take place in locations other than his bedroom).

A scene is reorganized by the process of *goal collection.* Goal-based expectations delimit what MOPs or scenes are likely to be undertaken when a goal is to be satisfied. One way that such an expectation can fail is if the anticipated scene does not take place. When this occurs, the scene that was actually perceived must be compared with the scene that was under construction. If their goal basis is the same, which it should be under ordinary circumstances, a scene reorganization takes place. The two scenes are compared for common aspects. When found, those common aspects are treated as the fixed expectations of the scene. The elements that were different are treated as variables in the scene. By collecting common elements according to goals in this way, new, and more abstract scenes are built.

One problem here is whether to replace old scenes by new scenes. For example, the scene BEDROOM seems an appropriate generalization of CRIB, but should ROOM be abstracted from bedroom? Finding the most useful, high level of abstraction is thus a problem for scene reorganization. (This problem occurs elsewhere as well, see Rosch, 1978; Abbott and Black, 1981.) The answer depends upon common goals and the variety of scripts that are used to achieve those goals. If the number of scripts attached to a scene is only one, then the scene has been undergeneralized. If it is fifty, then it has ben overgeneralized. Fixing an exact number here should probably await experimental results. It is unlikely that all people have the same criteria however.

Generalized and universal scenes

The issue of scene generalization can be approached from a different perspective. Rather than ask what the bases for generalization are, we can ask questions about the bases of scenes. A great many scenes seem to fall into a neat division that reflects their role in a MOP. Is there any sense in talking about a set of universal scenes that are derived from a universal MOP?

Nearly every MOP that we have described so far has been able to make use of scenes that were used by some other MOP. For example, we might ask how hotels are like airplanes, or how restaurants are like offices. On the surface, these entities do not seem all that much alike. But, M-HOTEL and M-AIRPLANE both share the scene CHECK-IN. M-RESTAURANT shares PAY-CASHIER with M-HOTEL. M-RESTAURANT shares ORDER with M-STORE.

This sharing of scenes is not random. With respect to physical and societal scenes, there really aren't all that many possibilities for what can be a scene. One of the reasons that people learn as well as they do is that they do not have an impossibly large number of structures to work with. Instead, they are constantly using the same structures over and over again. To put this another way, people wish to see new things in terms of what they have already seen. Thus, the resultant understanding of a new situation will be in terms of the original situation, with some variation. Now, it is possible to see the second item processed as really being radically different from the original item that it was being compared to. And, when such distinctions are maintained, memory structures remain highly idiosyncratic. But, sometimes it is advantageous to preserve initial generalities. Working from a few unique scenes, and viewing new items in terms of those scenes, will allow a great deal of power in generalization.

It is important then, that we attempt to somehow delimit what the range of scenes is. As we try to escape from the confines of the specific scene we find ourselves looking at two structures. The first of these is the scene that has broken away from specific contexts and are abstractions of what is generally true of any particular scene. These we will refer to as Generalized Scenes. At an even higher level of abstraction, however, we find a somewhat different set of scenes. These are scenes that contain no context information whatsoever, and are defined only in terms of the kinds of roles that they play in MOP structures. These scenes, which exist at the highest level of abstraction in memory, we shall call Universal Scenes. Together these scenes account for a fairly large number of the scenes that we use in MOPs.

It follows from the principles we have been developing that these two types of abstract scenes must exist. If understanders always attempt to abstract commonalities and index differences, then one consequence is that the abstraction process will continue as far as possible. Hence, we will find some structures in memory at this extreme level of generality. These will be the generalized scenes. We will also find structures at the highest level generality, that is, higher than generalized scenes. These will be the universal scenes. Thus we see then, that two sets of abstract scenes exist. One type contains generalizations within a context, and the other, generalizations that are role-related but context-free.

If you want to achieve a goal in a societal context, there are often a set of preliminary steps that have to be followed; a set of conditions that must be met at the time that the goal is about to be achieved; and a set of follow up actions that must be performed to undo some of the preliminaries and in general to wind things up. This basic pattern is exploited by people in their storage and learning capabilities, and it is this pattern that accounts for the use of universal scenes.

That such a set of universal scenes must exist follows from our need to abstract and generalize. For every event, we are attempting to find how that event relates to our general knowledge (e.g., how a new script can be inferred that colors the scene we are in). At the same time, we are attempting to collect similar specific knowledge in general, abstract, structures. Thus it follows that any scene should have a higher level, more abstract scene that it *colors*. This hierarchical organization, long exploited in Artificial Intelligence programs for concepts, has a realization in episodic structures as well. The question is simply, "What are the structures?"

There exist both generalized and universal scenes. At the highest level of abstraction, let us consider these eight universal scenes:

PREPARATORY
ENABLEMENT
PRECONDITION
SIDE-CONDITION
ACTION
POST-CONDITION
DISENABLEMENT
REALIZATION or TRANSITION

Of course, there is nothing immutable about how one must abstract and generalize. Nevertheless, the above scenes can be used to represent our abstract knowledge at the highest levels. Put together as a MOP, what we have is an abstraction of all MOPs that expresses the commonality that tends to hold between scenes in a MOP. It is, in a sense, the Universal MOP. We know, as understanders of the world around us, that whatever goal-oriented event we choose to process or recall, it is likely that it shares to some extent the structure (that is, the above scenes in the order presented) of this Universal MOP. The value of the Universal MOP in processing is simply that when all else fails, we can rely upon our knowledge of what goes on at the highest levels of generality to help us figure out what might be going on.

Let us now look at a few of the MOPs we have discussed from this perspective:

	PREP	ENABLE	PRECOND	SIDECOND	ACTION	POST-COND	DISENABLE	COMMENCI
U-MOP:								
M-RESTAU-RANT:	RESERVE	[go]	WAITING AREA	ORDER SERVE	[EAT]	PAY	[go]	
M-AIRPLANE:	RESERVE	[go]	CHECK-IN WAITING AREA	BAGGAGE BOARD	[FLY]	DEPLANE	BAGGAGE	DO
M-POV:	RESERVE	[go]	CHECK-IN WAITING AREA		[SERVICE]	PAY	CHECK-OUT [go]	

In the above diagram we can see that certain scenes appear quite frequently in the three MOPs illustrated. Moreover, these scenes play the same role with respect to their MOP in each case. The consequence of this is that we can anticipate the development, by any understanding system, of a set of generalized scenes that are useful in developing a rudimentary understanding of any new situation. Generalized scenes are activated in much the same way as regular scenes. During processing, if a MOP does not contain any scene information at a given point, the processor moves to the universal scene that is relevant and searches for a generalized scene that might be of some use. Thus if no specific scene is available for processing, the best generalized scene is used to aid in processing. As in processing with a regular scene, any information acquired in a generalized scene affects the scene regardless of what MOP was being served by that scene at the moment.

For example, CHECK-IN is a generalized scene that relates to the universal scene, PRECONDITION. When one is on one's first plane trip, and has not yet built a MOP structure to handle the situation, the scene for checking in one's baggage does not yet exist. The universal scene PRE-CONDITION, however is activated as a default from the universal MOP. From PRECONDITION one can move down to the more context oriented CHECK-IN and use it to handle the processing of the airport situation. At this point we might expect that CHECK-IN would continue to exist as a generalized scene, from which more specific scripts relating to hotels and airports as instantiations of CHECK-IN would be hung.

The disadvantage in such a system lies in the possibility of confusions. That is, as many different memories are stored under a single general structure, it becomes more and more difficult to tell them from one another. Look again at our person in the airport. If he lost his passport on a trip, he might try to recall when he last had it. The CHECK-IN scene is a likely candidate. But it is shared by both M-AIRPORT and M-HOTEL. It might be difficult to sort out the specifics of one experience from the other. Of course, as both scenes employ different scripts, separating one experience from the other is certainly possible. Nevertheless, there would be confusions caused by expectations copied directly from the scene that are uncolored. This is the price we pay for being able to generalize from one experience to the other. The advantage of the scheme however, is that the number of possible scenes is strictly limited by employing such generalized scenes. This helps us to learn, generalize, and limit memory searches.

Thus the MOPs that we have been discussing can be seen in relationship to each other. RESERVE and WAITING AREA can be seen as sharing a large amount of information wherever they are employed and allow for learning that occurs in one MOP to be applied in another. The advantage of this is obvious. If one wants to, one can see identity and learn across contexts. Nothing is lost, since differences can be indexed, and scripts created, that capture the particular aspects of a situation. Thus if it is useful to view a waiting room in a dentist's office and a waiting area in an airport as the same, a mechanism (a structure in this case) must be available for doing that. Certainly, the first time an airplane waiting area is encountered, if knowledge about dentists' waiting rooms is available, it would be helpful to use it. As we have said, we process what we experience to the closest possible episode we have in memory. Later, we may choose to ignore the similarities we found useful. But we also may continue to use such generalized scenes.

Not all scenes fit into this universal scheme. However, those that do provide the opportunity to know what the overall role of that scene is. Knowing that a scene has *enablement* as its purpose can allow us to know how to circumvent it or fix it if it fails. Thus, knowing things about the role of a scene (that is, its relationship to the universal scene that is its highest abstraction) tells us why that scene is around, which is useful when problems occur. Such knowledge also helps in initial processing when a *first approximation* is needed.

Other universal MOPs

A scene can be generalized if its role with respect to a MOP is standard. MOP-relatedness is a key issue in noting that CHECK-IN in M-HOTEL is the same as CHECK-IN in M-AIRPORT. But there are other aspects of many scenes that can relate them for the purposes of generalization. Likewise there are other universal MOPs that control these relations between scenes. One of these has to do with their contractual nature.

Consider PAY as a scene. We pay for airplanes before we use them, but we pay for restaurants and hotels afterwards. We pay for doctors and lawyers a long time afterwards. Thus, in terms of the Universal MOP discussed above, each of these PAYs has a different role. It is a precondition in some cases and a postcondition in others. Nevertheless, we certainly see PAY similarly in each case.

Now consider an agreement between friends, say an exchange of favors. It is not unreasonable for a person who has had trouble with a friend who did not pay back money owed to become uncertain about an agreement to exchange favors. Certainly this person can be expected to recall that his friend reneged on a previous agreement.

There seems to be something going on here that allows us to make appropriate generalizations on the basis of the role of a scene in a contractual relationship. The Universal MOP generalized the performance relations between scenes. In other words, it dealt with the temporal relationships between PAY and ORDER for example, in terms of their physical realizations of the steps towards the achievement of a goal. We might expect therefore, that other Universal MOPs (henceforth U-MOPs) relate to societal and personal MOPs. Thus, the Universal MOP that we referred to above, we shall rename UM-PERFORMANCE since it is not the only U-MOP. The role of UM-PERFORMANCE is to put together scenes in terms of their temporal sequence. The societal U-MOP (UM-AGREE-MENT) relies not upon the order in which actions are performed but rather upon viewing scenes as part of an agreement.

We introduce the U-MOP:UM-AGREEMENT which looks as follows:

UM-AGREEMENT:MAKE CONTRACT + MAKE ARRANGE-
MENTS + AGREE TO PERFORM + PERFORM-(ACTOR1)
+ PERFORM-(ACTOR2)

UM-AGREEMENT covers bets, signed contracts, trades of services, professional services, and agreements between people in general. In most circumstances that involve people in societal situations UM-AGREEMENT and UM-PERFORMANCE are operating, in the sense that they underlie the actual MOPs that are operating. In other words, we are always doing something in an episode, and, if it involves another person, we can be expected to have evoked a (possibly implicit) agreement that covers our actions.

The personal U-MOP is also usually operating in societal situations. This is UM-FIX-PROBLEM. It looks as follows:

UM-FIX-PROBLEM: DETERMINE PROBLEM + FINDFIXER
+ AGREE TO FIX + FIX + GRATITUDE

AGREE-TO-FIX and FIX are often filled by UM-PERFORMANCE and UM-AGREEMENT. Thus, visiting to a doctor's office involves UM-PERFORMANCE and UM-AGREEMENT as well as UM-FIX-PROBLEM. The reason UM-FIX-PROBLEM is present is that it establishes the role of the actor as a supplicant of sorts. In other words, a doctor is not only a professional provider of services (for which he is paid and thus requires no thanks) but he is also a fixer of problems (which does require thanks). We do not feel beholden to a restaurant for feeding us or an airline for taking us somewhere because we do not view them as having personally decided to help us with our problem. When things are impersonal, UM-FIX-PROBLEM is not in the picture. But personal exchanges cause us to view things slightly differently.

U-MOPs illustrate the fact that a given event can be viewed in a myriad of ways. Paying someone can be seen as the physical act of handing over money; as part of a precondition to service; as part of an agreement; and as part of an expression of gratitude. This ability to view something in alternate ways has profound implications for memory. Since, according to our views, processing and storage involve the same mechanisms, processing something in a different way implies storing it and being able to recall it only in that way. Thus, *paying* can be stored in any or all of the four different ways suggested above (and probably more). Here again, we see the trade-off between the power of generalization and learning and the potential for recall confusions.

To be specific when you check out of a hotel, the scenes CHECK-OUT and PAY are both operating. In addition, if something special were done for you GRATITUDE might be operating as well.

One confusion that may exist here has to do with our procedures. We have used PERFORM-(ACTOR2) as a generalized scene name for UM-AGREEMENT. PERFORM-(ACTOR2) refers to the second of the two acts agreed to in UM-AGREEMENT. Often PERFORM-(ACTOR2) is realized as PAY. In UM-PERFORMANCE we have a scene called POSTCONDITION. But, we referred to CHECK-OUT as the generalized scene. CHECK-OUT is, of course, a specialization of POSTCONDITION as is PAY a specialization of PERFORM2. That is, CHECK-OUT is to POSTCONDITION as *$HOTEL-CHECK-OUT* is to CHECK-OUT. That is, it copies over its identical parts and colors the rest with specifics that vary from the generalized norm. When a person is checking out of a hotel, he will use information from, and store memories connected with, expectation failures in any one of the three places: the script; the generalized scene; or the universal scene. In this case the scene CHECK-OUT is a generalized scene. Although it is quite general (it incorporates CHECK-OUT from M-SUPERMARKET and CHECK-OUT from M-RESTAURANT it is also a specialized form of the more general POSTCONDITION.

Thus, we are proposing two different types of generalizations with respect to scenes. The first, a generalized scene, is an attempt to gather together like information at a high level of abstraction, but with a significant amount of contextually-based information present nevertheless. The second, a Universal scene, is intended to represent the highest level of abstraction available, with no context-dependent information available. As we have continually insisted, there is no *correct* set of structures. As understanders we strive to store information at the level of specificity that will best allow us to access and use this information in the future. When no new information is available from an experience or where that information is of great general relevance, we attempt to store it as generally as possible. When, however, information is deemed to be of interest and is germane only to the memories currently being processed, we store that information as specifically as possible. Thus, information about ORDERing for example, can be stored in three places. We know certain things about it from its universal scene (PRECONDITION), and we also know specific things about it from its appropriate script (e.g., *$RESTAURANT-ORDER*). But, its most generally useful aspect is what is stored in ORDER itself, which is, in our new view, a generalized scene.

How it all works

Now consider a man who goes to the doctor, a restaurant, a supermarket, an auto parts store and has a plumber and a carpenter visit his home to make repairs. What structures in memory will he have used to process what went on during this busy day? Assuming that most everything proceeded in an ordinary way, without expectation failure, we would claim that three U-MOPs were used, namely:

> UM-AGREEMENT
> UM-PERFORMANCE
> UM-FIX-PROBLEM

Further, we would claim the following MOPS were used:

> M-RESTAURANT
> M-STORE
> M-PROF-HOME-VISIT
> M-PROF-OFFICE-VISIT

The question we wish to answer is, what scenes were used and how does memory appear at the end of this day? That is, what was stored where, what could have gotten confused with what, and what information would have been found where during processing?

One thing to note here is that certain experiences look similar from some points of view, yet are different from others. In other words, we can generalize from things in different ways. For example, the MOPs M-PROF-OFFICE-VISIT and M-PROF-HOME-VISIT control the doctor and the plumber experience respectively. From one point of view they are not at all similar. The first involves going to the doctor's office, checking in, waiting in the outer office, and so on, while the other involves no travel, waiting at home, and showing the plumber where in the house the problem is. From this point of view, they are not very similar (despite their names). From another point of view these experiences do have an important similarity. Namely, both the doctor and plumber experiences are aspects of UM-FIX-PROBLEM. Thus conclusions about a problem that was weighing on our hero's mind and that was alleviated by a professional, would apply in each case. We can see then, that by looking at events in terms of the different MOP structures that control our understanding of those events, we can develop new views of those structures and notice similarities that do not exist otherwise.

We see another example in the case of the restaurant and the auto-parts store. If our hero had trouble getting what he wanted in each place, some recall confusion might result, since both share ORDER. The poten-

EXPERIENCES

STRUCTURES	Restaurant	Auto parts store	Supervision needed	Doctor	Plumber	Carpenter
ORDER	✓	✓				
POST-COND: RAY	✓	✓	✓	?	?	?
GRATITUDE				✓	✓	
[go]	✓	✓	✓	✓		
WAITING AREA	✓			✓		
AGREE TO PERFORM DELIVER				✓	✓	✓
WAIT AT HOME					✓	✓
M-CONTRACT	✓			✓	✓	✓
UM-FIXPROBLEM				✓	✓	✓
M-HOUSECARE					✓	✓
M-EATING	✓		✓			
UM-PERFORMANCE	✓	✓	✓	✓		
PRECOND: WAIT	✓	✓		✓	✓	✓
$PAY	✓	✓	✓			

Figure 4

tial for confusion, and hence learning, across this set of experiences, is illustrated by the chart in Figure 4.

This chart reflects some of the commonalities here. We expect that our hero could get confused in some respects about what happened to him in which situation. In some of these situations he was going somewhere to do something. In others he had someone visit him. In some, he was part of a contract, which involved asking someone to fix a problem of his. Sometimes he has to wait at home or in a waiting area. We could go on and on here. The point is that different similarities occur when we view things at the level of Universal UNIVERSAL MOPs, Universal scenes and generalized scenes. At the level of scripts, except for [go] and some of the possible realizations of PAY, each story was quite different. But the doctor visit has something in common with the plumber visit (UM-FIX-PROBLEM) while the plumber visit is quite like the carpenter visit [UM-FIX-PROBLEM + M-PROFHOME VISIT].

The multiple levels of description available here allow for each of the commonalities and differences to be expressed. Our hero can use what he knows about POSTCONDITIONS, or PAY, or *$PAY*, or all three, to help him each time the matter comes up. What he learns from each experience can be applied at the level that is most appropriate. Here again, the price of learning is memory confusion.

Summary

Universal MOPs organize universal scenes. MOPs organize generalized scenes. Universal scenes point to generalized scenes, which color them. Generalized scenes point to scripts, which color them. Any experience will be processed, in part, by episodic information attached to each of these structures and will affect each of the structures that helped in the processing.

10   Indexing and search

In any discussion of memory, the ultimate problem is indexing. When one memory reminds us of another, we have done two things. First, for a variety of processing reasons, we have found a memory structure. Second, we have found, via some indexing method, the particular place in that structure where the specific memory of which we were reminded was stored. We have previously investigated two questions about memory structures:

1. How was the particular structure found?
2. What are the range and nature of such structures?

These questions apply to indices within structures as well. We must know how to find indices and what the nature of an index is.

Failed expectations are a critical part of our memory organization procedures. They represent a first attempt at indexing. Of course, indexing is not a purpose which causes an expectation to fail. An expectation is tried (and fails) for processing reasons, and its failure must be explained for processing reasons. In order to understand what is happening, we make expectations and attempt to explain expectation failures when they occur.

But what happens after an expectation failure has been explained? Failed expectations must be re-examined. Memory structures must be altered. Old ones must be changed, new ones created and, most significantly, new memories must be stored.

All three of these processes depend upon indexing. The use of memory for understanding also depends upon indexing, but that phase is simply a user of indexing rather than a creator of indexing. In initial understanding, we find memories by noting the right structures and indices, and then using that information to search memory.

Thus there are the following issues:

1. During the initial understanding phase, how are memory structures, and indices inside those memory structures, decided upon for search?

158

2. How do failed expectations help us find new indices for storing the memories connected to those failed expectations?
3. How does the use of indexing cause new memory structures to be created?
4. How is a new episode stored in memory, i.e., how are the indices chosen for storage purposes?

What can be an index

We have examined a number of reminding examples that would seem to bear upon the issue of what can be an index. We will reconsider some of them here. Before we do that however, it is important to make a point about the nature of indices in general. Indices depend upon the structures they index for their existence. The *correct set* of indices in any system depend upon what is deemed significant by that system. A library is a good example of a system that employs indexing. No library indexing system uses, so far as we are aware, the color of a book as one of its indices. Bookstores use *publishers* as an index so they can order from them. Libraries do not use *publishers* as an index made available to the public in the card catalogue.

The reason for all this seems simple enough. An index indicates what is deemed significant for the purpose of the structure that employs that index. The same ought to be true of any human memory indexing scheme. That is, what will serve as a good index is something that is structure-dependent. To put this more concretely, we should not expect that what will make a good index in a given TOP, will be of use in a given MOP, or even that the indices of one MOP relate significantly to those of another MOP. An index within a structure should be a function of the most important aspects that helped to define that structure in the first place. Thus, indexing is vitally related to the alteration and creation of structures.

Since indices are related to the significant aspects that define a structure, it follows that we must examine the basis of a structure to consider what its indices might be. With that in mind, let's consider some structures and associated indices.

Indexing in TOPs

In Chapters 4 and 7, we presented some reminding examples that we argued were accounted for by the fact that they utilized the same TOP structure and had an identical set of indices. Let's examine the indices in some of those examples more closely.

Consider again case J, the story about the dieting woman who, after

forcing her choice of restaurant because of her diet, then ordered food
differently than she had said she would. There, we suggested that the
structure that handled these cases was CG;CS(Competing Goal; Compromise Solution). We further suggested that case K, the story about the
professor making an appointment with a student, was also handled by
CG;CS. Further, we claimed that a conversation about the Middle East
situation might also use CG;CS. We suggested that the indices for these were:

Case J	Case K	Mid-East
diet	feeling "had"	Mid-East
restaurant	reneged on	situation
feeling "had" reneged on promise	promise	Arab demands

A TOP has two basic parts, a goal expression and a condition that
relates to that goal. It is the role of indices to somehow further specify the
significant aspects of the structure they index. Hence, we would expect
that both **Competing Goal** and **Compromise Solution** ought to be further
specified by any indices used within the TOP CG;CS. We can look first at
the way in which the goal portion of the TOP can be further specified, and
used as indices.

Goal specification can be made through noting the general class of the
goal, the particular goal, or the object of the goal, defined at different
levels of description. So, we can specify a goal by noting that it is of a
certain class (satisfaction, achievement, etc), is itself a particular goal
(eat, own, go and so on), and is related to a particular goal *object,* (eat in
a *restaurant,* own a *car,* or go to *New York*). By further refining the
specification of the goal object, we can define and identify very particular
goals (e.g. eat in Leon's, or own a Maserati).

In CG;CS we don't just have a *goal,* we have a *competing goal,* and the
specification that we desire must be treated as a specification of the goal
competition itself. Thus, the next question to ask is what the area of
competition is. In case J, the competing goal is **restaurant selection.** That
is, the issue is not the general goal of eating, because that has been
agreed upon. They have also agreed at the next level of goal specification, namely, they have agreed to **eat in a restaurant.**

In a complex indexing scheme, such distinctions can be of crucial importance. We can see that the match between J and K has nothing to do with
eating or restaurants. K matched J in the fact that there was a goal object
selection problem. That is, there was a problem that existed in terms of the
selection of the goal object, **restaurant** in case J and **appointment time** in
case K. On the other hand, the two episodes in J match each other (from a
goal-related point of view) in **restaurant selection specification,** in that the

object of the goal in general, **restaurant,** had already been chosen and the problem was in terms of an even greater specification of this object. In other words, goal refinement and the abstraction of the process of goal refinement are a significant part of the indexing problem.

In general, when a goal is selected, the following specifications are made:

1. goal type (e.g. satisfaction)
2. goal action (e.g. eat)
3. goal object (e.g. eat lobster)
4. goal features (e.g. in a restaurant)

These four aspects can be further specified by a variety of particulars on the general type (e.g., a Maine lobster, or a particular restaurant).

In goal competition, the competition can manifest itself in a number of ways. It can involve any of the four aspects listed above, at varying levels of specification. Thus, two people can compete with respect to the activity to be pursued, where to pursue it, how much to spend, where to sit, and so on. In general, the competition can revolve around the selection of a particular choice to be agreed upon, or the mutual decision to go after identical objects in a goal that presumes that sharing is infeasible or undesired.

Our preliminary analysis of case J, as an instance of **restaurant selection specification** involved the uncritical use of *restaurant* as an index. However, any object in the world cannot be effectively used as an index for any structure. It is through the use of certain constraints on what can be an index that reminding is more likely to occur. Unconstrained indexing would result in few matches. In a TOP, goal specifications are permissible indices. In CG;CS in particular, specifications of the selection problem that caused the goal competition are not only permissible indices, they exemplify the principle upon which such indexing is based.

An index refines a memeory structure within the domain of that structure. For the goal competition domain, an index must specify the area of competition – in case J, *restaurant selection*. In case K, we have something like *time selection*. The fact that J reminded someone of K implies that these somehow match.

But how? In general, indices must both be from the same specification class. That is to say, they must match in terms of the four aspects of a goal mentioned above. It is unlikely that a story involving a disagreement on the selection of a goal activity would remind someone of a problem involving the selection of particular features of a goal object. Of course it is possible in principle. Indices behave in much the same way as MOPs, TOPs, and scenes, in that they change over time depending upon actual experience. A person who only had one disagreement (involving a goal competition) in his life, would certainly get reminded of that experience by another, regardless of whether the two episodes matched at the level we are discussing.

So, the question is, is this a match of the same kind? In case K, the disagreement is about the time of a meeting. Both this and **restaurant selection** are goal feature specifications. Both are cases of *selection of goal feature specification*. The implication here is that indices can match in two ways. First by identity, as was the case in the two episodes in case J. And, second, by being members of the same class of phenomenon, in this case *selection of goal feature specification*.

Thus, we see that our first assumptions about indexing have held true for goal competition. The type of goal specification, in this case specification of goals that are involved in a competition, can be used as a potential index. Further, we have a corollary rule for matching of indices – types of goal specifications can match by identity or by being members of the same class of specifications within a TOP. What other kinds of indices and matching rules are there?

The other proposed index in case J, **dieting,** is clearly a different kind of index than we had above. **Dieting** relates to the reason for the goal competition's existence. The assumption is that there would be no disagreement on the goal particulars if not for **dieting.** These two indices, **dieting** and what we shall now call **restaurant selection specification,** span the range of possible TOPs headed by *competition goals.* Namely, what we have is:

1. an area of disagreement
2. a reason for the disagreement

These two subjects are the basis for refinements that act as indices within the **competition goal** part of CG;CS.

There are a large set of possibilities for why there might be a goal competition in a given situation. Nevertheless, most reasons have a logic to them. Dieting is, after all, related to **eat,** the dominating goal in case J. Certainly if *dieting* were given as the reason for the disagreement in case K, it would seem quite odd.

The implication is then, that the *reason for a goal competition* is dependent on the particulars of the disagreement, and hence cannot function as an independent index. For example, in case J, *dieting* is not an independent index, but rather is stored in terms of **restaurant selection.** Therefore, it will not be found unless an initial match on the particulars of the disagreement, **restaurant-selection,** has been made.

We now move over to the condition part of CG;CS, namely **compromise solution.** Clearly, aspects of a compromise are potential indices of it. A compromise consists of roughly three parts: the two original, and diverging, positions and an agreed-upon third position. And, just as the two initial positions have a reason to justify them, the third agreed upon solution has a complex reason (usually the amalgamation of the two initial reasons) behind it.

Cases J and K involve expectations generated by the compromise which are subsequently confounded. And, as we have said, explanations of expectation failures can be indices in a structure. In this case, we do not have an explanation, but there is an analysis of the expectation failure: the reason given that justified compromise was invalidated by one of the participants.

The index for both episodes in case J and the one in case K then is: *CG;CS: compromise failure – analysis: reason invalid.* In other words, CG;CS carries with it an expectation that there will be a reason behind the compromise. The **compromise solution** aspect to CG;CS consists of three parts, each of which contributes to the creation of an expectation in CG;CS. Expectations can be traced to their origins. The origins differ according to the structure that generated them. Thus, within CG;CS, there will be indices corresponding to various expectations about compromising. Expectation failures may be analyzed according to reasons then. Here, *actor's reason invalid* is an index to one of those expectations. Earlier we used specification of the goal and its related objects as an index into a TOP, now we have found a second kind of index into these structures, namely, the analyses of expectation failures.

The last index in cases J and K is *feeling had.* This is an index that depends upon an affect that results from the experience indexed by CG;CS itself and not from one of its parts. Since the feelings were the same in each case, the index is simply what we said it was. The third type of indexing then is based on the rule that – in a TOP, a feeling that follows after the episode is completed, can be an index in that TOP.

Thus, upon a reanalysis of the indices in case J and case K, we find:

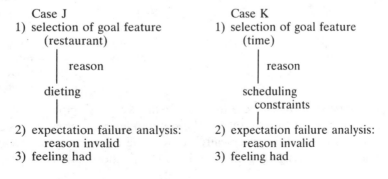

Case J
1) selection of goal feature
   (restaurant)

   | reason

   dieting
   |
2) expectation failure analysis:
   reason invalid
3) feeling had

Case K
1) selection of goal feature
   (time)

   | reason

   scheduling
   constraints
   |
2) expectation failure analysis:
   reason invalid
3) feeling had

The two episodes in J share identical indices. Case K is identical except for the particular specification of the goal feature (restaurant vs. time). The fact that the reasons are different follows from the initial difference between the goal features and is thus irrelevant.

Now consider the case of the Middle East example. If, as we claim, the organizing TOP in this case is also CG;CS, we are obligated, since indices are structure-dependent, to consider what other indices might be relevant here.

According to the scheme proposed above, *Middle East situation* is an unrealistic index because of its generality. However, it is possible to construct a realistic index with the same content. The Middle East situation is a problem because there is a competition goal involving the same goal object (Palestine) being pursued by two different parties. So, one index, derived from the CG part of CG;CS, is a particular goal object that cannot be jointly possessed (or at least that is assumed by the participants in the goal conflict). Thus, the indexing scheme suggested for CG;CS seems general enough to apply in diverse situations.

Some more indices for TOPs

Now let's consider some of the other TOPs, discussed in Chapter 7, which we reproduce here:

REMINDING	GOAL	CONDITIONS	FEATURES
R&J/West Side Story	Mutual goal pursuit	Outside opposition	Young lovers; false report of death
R&J/Back Street	Mutual goal pursuit	Outside opposition	Explanation: next time inform co-planner
Munich/ Afghanistan	Possession goal	Evil intent	Countries; invasions
Nixon/ Mayor of New Haven	Achieve power position	Presence of enemies	Political office; campaign promises

To what extent does the indexing scheme we have employed in CG;CS have to be altered to account for the remindings mentioned in this chart?

To put this question specifically, what is the relationship of the indices used above in MG;OO, PG;EI, and AS;UP to those TOPs? Further, we would like to explore the possibility that there are some general principles available for indexing TOPs.

In MG;OO, we used three indices: young lovers, false report of death, and an explanation (next time inform co-planner). As before, let's consider the goal-oriented aspect separately from the condition. When we listed the possible goal aspects to be specified in CG:CS, we clearly left out an important aspect – characteristics of the actors in the goal pursuit. Just as with the characteristics of the goal object, it is reasonable to expect that characteristics of the actors involved in pursuing the goal will serve as indices in a TOP. Thus, we have a fourth type of index – specifications as to particulars relating to the actors pursuing a goal.

It follows from the above then, that there is an index in the *Romeo and Juliet* story that we didn't mention, namely, the particulars of the goal. In this case, the goal being pursued is a love relationship between the actors. This is an obvious match with *West Side Story*.

Now, what about the false report of death? This relates to the condition part of the TOP. As before, the condition, in this case Outside Opposition, has aspects that naturally lend themselves to further specification for the purposes of indexing. Thus, Outside Opposition has actors, their goals, the reasons for those goals, their actions, the effects of those actions, and conclusions to be drawn from the experience. More than one of these aspects of the condition matches between *Romeo and Juliet* and *West Side Story*. The actors who constitute the outside opposition are the families of the actors involved in the goal pursuit. The effect of their opposition also matches – in this case driving the lovers to surreptitious means of getting together. The *false report of death* is a consequence of the planners' reaction to the outside oppostion. The actual death of the hero is the end result. Further, the same conclusion should be drawn – *next time inform co-planner*. This is used in the *Back Street* reminding as well.

There are two essential points to be made. First, there is a systematic way to account for indexing. It has to do with aspects of the goal pursuit in the goal part of a TOP, and with the details of the conditions. The types of goal-related indices are invariant across TOPs. The same goal aspects are generally relevant. Of course, certain unique aspects of the particular goal being pursued will add some more possibilities for indices. The indices relevant to the conditions of a TOP depend upon the conditions themselves. The potential indices are provided by the fillers of the Conceptual Dependency slots (see Schank, 1972; 1975) that describe the conditions in detail. That is, it is the meaning of Outside Opposition, that provides the potential set of indices.

The second point is that if you look in a systematic way, it is clear that

in remindings, the event that evoked the reminding and the event that
was called up have the potential to match in many ways. In the case of
the *Romeo and Juliet* and *West Side Story* match we find a great many
more than two indices already mentioned. They match on:

> actor of goal pursuit
> goal object
> actor of outside opposition
> the reasons for the outside opposition
> the actions of these actors
> the effects of their actions
> the consequences of the reaction to the opposition
> the end results

By taking into consideration all these aspects, we can write the following summary:

Yound lovers try to pursue their relationship. Their families object because they
are from different groups that dislike each other. The families try to keep them
apart. The young lovers plan to get around this. A false report of the death of the
woman is received by the man. He dies having lost all hope.

The key point here is that the above summary is natural, although it
leaves out the details. It isn't clear whether the summary is of *Romeo and
Juliet* or *West Side Story*. To put this another way, a plot outline can
consist of particular indices in a TOP filled in with identical semantic
content.

It is not necessary to belabor the general point of indexing TOPs.
Hence, we shall not get into the details of the three other TOPs mentioned above. With little effort, it can be seen that the same general
principles apply. Thus, we have:

TOP INDEXING

In a TOP, indices are constructed by giving the particulars of the slots in a goal
pursuit and the particulars of the conditions. Each slot in the particulars of either,
or their combination, is a potential index.

From TOPs to MOPs

One issue that is worth discussing when we talk about indexing in TOPs is
the problem of how TOPs relate to MOPs. TOPs are context-independent
entities in that the goals, and conditions on goals, in TOPs have no relationship to particular scenes. Rather, TOPs relate to goals that transcend
scenes. But it is possible, considering what we have said about indices
that TOPs can, given the proper conditions, cause memory to create new
MOPs.

The indices mentioned earlier have a sequential flavor to them when they describe characteristic events that make up, for example **outside opposition** or **compromise solution.** That is, one could create a MOP that provided a sequence to a set of scenes that comprised **outside opposition.** The problem is that what we want to say or know about **outside opposition** applies whether we are talking about lovers plotting to marry, or a new building permit being requested. We need to know about **outside opposition** apart from its context, which is not possible using scenes based in particular contexts.

But suppose an understander were to see *Romeo and Juliet* first, then *West Side Story,* and then many more stories with roughly the same set of events. It would not be necessary for them to all end unhappily for someone, say a professional family counselor, to develop a MOP that corresponded to FAMILY OPPOSITION TO CHILD'S PLANS. Such a MOP would be comprised primarily of personal scenes such as PREVENT GET TOGETHER and PLAN SURREPTITIOUSLY.

The point is this. A MOP can be built when several episodes are understood in terms of a TOP by using the same indices. If the same indices keep recurring, a pattern is developing. Such a pattern must be recalled if an understander is to make sensible predictions. He can only do so by developing a new MOP to account for the pattern he has just noticed. Thus MOPs can be derived from TOPs whose indices are frequently repeated.

Building generalized scenes

Consider the hotel CHECK-IN scene. When you check in to a hotel for the first time, it is natural to build a physical scene corresponding to HOTEL-CHECK-IN that includes signing the register, getting the key, giving them your credit card and hotel key, having the bellhop take your luggage. But according to what we have expressed about generalized scenes, HOTEL-CHECK-IN should not exist in that form for long. It is important that HOTEL-CHECK-IN be compared to AIRPORT-CHECK-IN and that its commonalities be abstracted out. Ideally, we want HOTEL-CHECK-IN to become a script that colors the CHECK-IN scene. This is done by making reference to the template provided by the Universal MOP.

Every time a new scene is formed, it is compared against the Universal MOP with respect to its place in the overall structures of that MOP. This is a necessary factor in processing in that new scenes are created though the use of the very general Universal scene structures. In other words, since HOTEL-CHECK-IN is a precondition to the HOTEL-ROOM scene in M-HOTEL it is developed by and checked against the Universal PRECONDITION SCENE in the Universal MOP when it is first created.

In order for the check with the Universal MOP to bear fruit, it is necessary that previous scenes checked with it have been indexed in such a way that similar scenes will be similarly indexed. In the case under consideration, AIRPORT-CHECK-IN must be indexed in terms of the Universal MOP preconditions scene using the same index or indices that will be used for HOTEL-CHECK-IN, if they are to match against each other and form a generalized scene. What might this identical index or indices be?

Here are some possibilities:

> money-related
> sealing with management of some organization
> precondition to service by large organization
> invoices, documents
> big desk with employee behind it

Here again, we face the same problem we had in attempting to find some system in the seemingly random set of possible indices for TOPs. Is there any system available here?

Generalized scenes play much the same role in memory as TOPs. Generalized scenes serve to store together, in the same terms, information from different contexts that share like elements. For TOPs, these like elements are the common goals and conditions that temper the achievement of those goals. For generalized scenes, the commonality is the purpose of the interaction and the more or less standard behavior associated with actors and objects in standard contexts.

While there is great generality to be obtained by storing like things together, there is also a problem regarding the initial storage and subsequent retrieval of information stored in such a general scheme. In other words, generalized scenes need indices within them also.

Now let us look at what a full-blown generalized scene such as CHECK-IN would look like in a memeory that had many experiences. We presume that CHECK-IN is used by M-HOTEL and M-AIRPLANE. Where else is it used? Or, to put this another way – how is it that CHECK-IN became a generalized scene? These questions are closely related.

Consider the relationship of CHECK-IN to M-HOTEL and M-AIR-PLANE. What commonality does CHECK-IN express that allows it to function usefully in both MOPs?

Because CHECK-IN plays the role of PRECONDITION in the Universal MOP, its significance in each MOP is that it contains information relevant to management-defined preconditons for the use of some resource. Or to put it simply, CHECK-IN is what you have to do if you want to do an activity controlled by an organization. CHECK-IN has a number of purposes. It is initiated to establish the right of the actor to use the service of the organization. Since this right is often established by the payment of money, the establishment of identity, and so on, CHECK-IN's role is to provide relevant expectations about these situations.

Now, one question is – how do we find memories stored in terms of check-ins? A second question is – how did CHECK-IN develop? The answer to both these questions depends upon how indexing is accomplished in generalized scenes. Because the purpose of a generalized scene is to store together the aspects of a situation that have great commonality, it follows that the variance on that commonality are its potential indices. Keeping in mind that CHECK-IN is related to the PRECONDITIONS universal scene, and that we are dealing with preconditions for action by an institution, we can assemble a plausible list of the roles (and thus the indices) in such a scene with relative ease. They are the answers to the following questions:

Preconditions to service
    1.   Who is management?
    2.   What does management control?
    3.   What do they require for its use?
    4.   Why do they require it?
    5.   Who are the clients?
    6.   What props does the physical scene contain?

The actual indices in use are derived from the answers to these questions. Thus, *hotel, money, credit card,* or *passport,* and so on can serve as indices with CHECK-IN.

As we said earlier, HOTEL-CHECK-IN is matched against the PRECONDITION scene in the Universal MOP because it has the same precondition role. It is checked for its indices, which as we can now see, are roughly the answers to the questions above.

These seven answers form the basis for the storage of *$HOTEL-CHECK-IN* as part of CHECK-IN. CHECK-IN looks like this prior to the addition of *$HOTEL-CHECK-IN:*

> enter environment
> go to desk where representative of management is
> inform him of your purpose
> produce documents
> complete documents and transfer
> pay (often implicit)
> get informed of next location
> go to next location

Then the decision to hold HOTEL-CHECK-IN as a separate memory structure is made, HOTEL-CHECK-IN is compared against CHECK-IN and *$HOTEL-CHECK-IN* is created. It is created by indexing the differences between the generalized scene and the new scene. Thus, for example, **produce documents** is copied into *$HOTEL-CHECK-IN* as null since no documents are usually needed. **Transfer** is given an object (namely a key). Thus, *key* is used as an index to **transfer** by which *$HOTEL-CHECK-IN* is found.

Three important points about indexing are illustrated here:

> A: Expectation failures are more useful as indices in scripts, than as indices in generalized scenes.

To see this, let's consider **produce documents** again. It is reasonable not to have an expectation that documents are required in *$HOTEL-CHECK-IN*. But, in a foreign country, a passport is often required for checking into a hotel. In certain countries, a document indicating that you have registered with the police is often required. These exceptions could cause us to attempt to create a new script that would also be stored in terms of CHECK-IN. But, the commonality with the rest of *$HOTEL-CHECK-IN* is too strong. Hence, the sensible course of action is to mark the failure the first time it occurs. At that point, we have created an index that consists of the unexpected requirements to **produce documents** and adds **passport** and **police certificate** as indices to that failure.

The second indexing issue is:

> B: Indices can be used to find scripts (and particular episodes) in a scene.

When **key** or **elevator** is into the generalized scene CHECK-IN, *$HOTEL-CHECK-IN* comes quickly to mind. These indices help call in the right processing structure. Thus we can imagine something like "I was dealing with some papers over a big desk and they handed me a key – oh it must have been a hotel." Of course, it could have been a safe-deposit box in a bank too, but in a sense that's the point. Such things come to mind given the general description of the scene in the most neutral terms (the rudiments of CHECK-IN) and a prop from the specific instance (an index to the script stored in terms of that scene). Thus, indices point to scripts from generalized scenes. And,

> C: Once a script has been determined, it can be used to index its own colorations within the generalized scene that spawned it.

We have been discussing *C* a great deal without actualy mentioning it specifically. A script *colors* a scene by indexing every expectation from the scene through the script. In other words we have something like *transfer in the case of $HOTEL-CHECK-IN leads one to expect the key.* Thus, just as the seven questions above can lead one to *$HOTEL-CHECK-IN*, so *$HOTEL-CHECK-IN* can lead one to each of the answers.

Thus, the initial question of how a generalized scene continually develops is that new scenes are compared against it. If there is enough of a match, the generalized scene replaces the particular scene, which becomes a script, indexed under, and coloring, the generalized scene.

So, the answer to what indices are used in generalized scenes are those mentioned in A, B, and C above, which in turn depend upon the answer to a set of questions regarding the particulars of the actions described by the generalized scene.

Indexing other kinds of expectation failure

Not all expectations are straightforward. When the world does not conform to what we expected, it does not necessarily follow that what happened was unexpected. That is, we are not always attempting to predict anything and everything that might happen.

One of the most important points about an expectation is, as we have said, that it can fail. Expectations that succeed are boring. They are of use in processing, of course. They help us to make sense of the world around us. But, from the point of view of a developing memory, that is, one that makes new generalizations and learns, a successful expectation is of no help. A failed expectation, on the other hand, forces us to create indices to memories that exemplify that failure. Further encounters with those indexed memories, that is, repeated failures leading to repeated remindings, force us to alter our expectations.

The major problem is, of course, what to do when an expectation fails. Expectations brought together in one scene, when they fail, can be traced to the proper place in memory for an update of the most relevant memory structure. This allows us to modify that structure and learn from our experience.

Consider a person in a given situation. The scene in which he is operating supplies expectations relevant to that situation. (Of course, there is likely to be more than one operating scene at any one time. But we are attempting to keep things simple here.) This scene is being employed by some MOP. For example in a car we might have:

```
        M-TRAVEL
           |
          CAR
           |
 $DRIVE  $TALK  $ENJOY-SCENERY
```

Let us assume that there are three scripts active in this scene at the same time. Now suppose a car swerves out in front of the driver. The driver reacts almost by instinct. Clearly whatever he does is part of *$DRIVE* by definition. But, if his later analysis of what he did makes him feel uncomfortable in some way, for example if he believes that he usually reacts correctly in crisis situations, but here did not, this analysis will modify his memory. But what does it modify?

He was in *$DRIVE* at the time. The physical manifestation of the action he performed was encoded in *$DRIVE.* The act of reflecting upon what he did, however, belongs elsewhere. It should modify a MOP that encodes knowledge of one's behavior in a crisis. We can call that MOP M-CRISIS-SITUATION. We can modify that MOP by noting that the expectation that failed in *$DRIVE* was one that was of one's own behavior in a crisis. That is, knowing the kind of expectation that failed helps us to modify the right structure, and in this case one that was not obviously in operation at the time. Thus, we might expect our driver to consider drive more carefully because expectations formed earlier about his ability to react to crises seem to be no longer applicable. In other words, we can change our world view upon reflection. Thus some MOPs can be consciously modified.

Consider another example. A hotel room is clearly a scene. When the plaster falls on you in your bed in a hotel room, you have experienced a failure of some kind. You would like to modify your memory accordingly. But what does that involve? Here again, none of the MOPs that we would like to modify were necessarily active at the moment the plaster fell. Nevertheless, we would like to possibly do the following things (classified according to what the expectations involved were about):

OTHER PEOPLE
The person we are with might have reacted hysterically to the plaster falling. We would want to modify our expectations about that person for use in similar situations.

INSTITUTIONS
We might not want to use this hotel again or even this chain of hotels again. We then might want to record this experience in terms of the institution's view on maintenance. Perhaps if this hotel is owned by an airline, we might conclude that it is unsafe to fly that airline.

OUTSIDE EVENTS
If the plaster fell at a crucial moment, we might want to update a MOP containing information about sequences of events controlled by destiny that negatively affect us just when we think everything is going fine. Such expectations are of the "everything always happens to me" type.

OURSELVES
Here again, we might have expected that we would do something in this situation (complain, wake up) that we did not do. Again an update of the appropriate structure is required.

Making these modifications requires establishing what structures are relevant. Expectations that fail directly are easy to trace to an appropriate structure. But we can just not add an expectation to the hotel room scene that plaster will fall on our heads in bed in a hotel. We also do not expect that some particular hotel is shabby or that our companion may be hysterical. None of these are failed expectations in the straightforward sense of that term. That is we didn't generate an expectation and then see it fail. Rather, something happened for which we had no expectation but which nevertheless contradicts what we would have predicted if we had been forced to predict. We call this situation Non-initiated Expectation Failure. (It is similar to Non-Initiated Goal Frustration (NIGF) that we discussed in Schank & Abelson, 1977.)

Beyond failures

The concept of failure alone is not sufficient to explain expectation modification or reminding. Further, the word *failure* can be confusing. We remember a great many things, not only seeming failures. It might seem more reasonable to say that we remember what is unusual in some way, while failing to be able to recall the mundane. But *unusual* is a difficult concept to define. We have concentrated on failed expectations as the basis for reminding and memory organization. *Unusual* is then defined in this sense: any event that differs significantly from our expectation is unusual. That difference should be remembered if it has potential processing value. Potential processing value is determined by storing the difference temporarily until reminding calls the unusual event into play. By *failed*, then, we do not mean *negative event*. Goals should not be confused with expectations.

How then can an expectation fail? On the surface an expectation can either succeed or fail. That is, either what we expected happened or it did not. This is the simple case. It is relevant in all situations whether or not there was some goal operating. But there is no goal operating only when we are passively observing the world around us. It might seem that there is no goal operating when we are observing other people's behavior and have absolutely no interest in the outcome. But even then often there is a goal operating, since whatever goal that they are pursuing, although we may not care about them achieving it, may be one we desire to achieve at some future time. Thus, their good or bad plan might be worth observing. So the simple observation that an expectation has failed is simply not enough. We must take the relevant goals that are operating into account. It is the success and failure of goals that are the raison d'etre of our understanding systems. Thus, it is likely that we will index a failed expectation by the relationship of that failure to the success or failure of any goal that might be involved.

Given that, consider the following combinations of expectations and goals:

> given expectation E0 that X will happen;
> and Goal G that the actor wants;
> and expectation E1 that X will lead to G;
> and expectation E2 that G will make you happy;
> and expectation E3 that no other goals will be satisfied if X happens.

If what actually happens is called Y, we have the following possibilities:

0. E0 fails; G fails
1. E0 fails; G succeeds
2. E0 fails; Y partially satisfies G
3. E0 fails; Y is better than X at satisfying G
4. E0 succeeds (Y=X) but E1 fails; (thus G remains unsatisfied)
5. E0 fails; G=Y; (Y turns out to satisfy G)
6. E0 succeeds; E1 succeeds; E2 fails; (G wasn't what was wanted)
7. E0 succeeds; E1, E2, succeed; but E3 fails; (you got more than just G)

The above situations regarding expectations can be summarized as follows:

0. Failure
1. Lucky Success
2. Partial Success
3. More Than You Had Hoped
4. Bad Plan
5. Unexpected Success
6. Not Knowing One's Own Mind
7. Success Beyond One's Dreams

It might seem that what we have listed above are sometimes failures and sometimes not. Actually they are all failures. That is, as understanders we create expectations about what will happen. When those expectations are wrong, when what we thought would happen does not, it is necessary to revise our internal structures to take the error into account. If we do not learn from our successes as well as our failures we are not behaving intelligently. But a success that went exactly according to plan is not one that needs to be learned from. The knowledge that should be applied in the future with respect to the successful goal was already there prior to that successful experience. It is unexpected success, or success by unexpected means, that involves expectation failure, and hence has the greater potential for learning.

We have a great many levels of expectation active at any given moment. Take, for example, the simple act of ordering in a restaurant. We expect a menu, but that could fail. We expect that we will get what we ordered, but that could fail. We expect that what we ordered will taste good, but that could fail. We expect that having eaten what tasted good we will be satisfied, but that could fail.

Each of these are expectations about the same event, but at different levels, focusing on different aspects. The menu is an expectation about preconditions for an action. Getting what we ordered is an expectation about the results of an action. Liking what we ordered is an expectation about a low level goal dominating our action. Feeling satisfied is an expectation that comes from a higher level goal dominating the lower level goal.

Each of these expectations is present at the time when we look for the menu. Failures in any of these expectations would need to be recorded so that we could learn from whatever mistake occurred. Each expectation failure would need to be explained.

For example, we might want to record in our memories for each case above:

> Menu – don't look for a menu in a fast food place, they don't have them
> Order – be careful to say what you want loudly here, the waitress is hard of hearing
> Like – don't order the roast beef here
> Satisfied – remember that one portion is never enough on Tuesdays after you have lectured

A crucial problem here is determining where the newly learned rule derived from the expectation failure must be placed. For example, above we can learn about that particular restaurant, restaurants in general, or about ourselves. The proper place for the new expectation rule depends partly on where the expectation came from in the first place, and partly on the nature of the explanation that accounted for the failure.

Indexing by explanation

One of the possible results of expectation failure is the creation of new memory structures. But this is not always the most desirable course of action. Sometimes it is best to alter little. Not every expectation failure should necessarily cause us to modify generalized memory structures. The first time an expectation failure occurs it may be best to simply record the specific episode that caused the failure, indexed by the failed expectation and an explanation of the failure.

Thus, we must create an explanation of the expectation failure. Ideally the explanation should be at the most general possible level. In the examples of reminding cited in Chapters 3 and 4, the explanations of expectation failure were always more general than the particular situation. Thus, we are not reminded only of steak-cooking when the server fails to cook the meat correctly. Similarly, we are reminded of a certain kind of planning failure in The Walking Aunt, not of problems related to walking home. It is clear then, that expectation failures, to be most useful in learning, should cause us to modify our expectations in a general way.

The problem of creating explanations for expectation failures requires us to first:

1. Establish what expectation failed, i.e., what exactly was it an expectation about?
2. Find the memory structure that generated the expectation
3. Establish the type of failure that it was, i.e., which of the above seven types was involved?

Once we have established, for example, that the failure was one that involved somebody's action in pursuit of a plan, we can attempt to explain the failure. The resultant explanation is about why a different thing occurred from what was expected at a given point in a memory structure. That explanation is independent of the particular context in which the failure occurred (e.g., steak-cooking), but not of the memory structure involved (e.g., M-PROVIDE-SERVICE and the SERVE scene). The new explanation is then used as an index in SERVE. Since SERVE is a generalized scene, and thus relatively abstract, learning has occurred across contexts. That is, this explanation, which was found relevant for a particular situation, has now been stored in a very general memory structure in a very general way. It will thus be useful for reminding and the eventual alteration of the structure. This can occur when the same explanation is conjured up again for a different situation in the same memory structure.

Thus, our last class of indices used for MOPs, generalized scenes, and scripts, are explanations of failure. These indices are constructed at the most general level of explanation possible, as determined by tracking the expectation failure to its source.

Indexing and initial understanding

Now that we have seen what indices are like and how they work, we return to the question of how indices are used in the initial understanding phase. When an input is first processed, the following questions are (unconsciously, of course) asked. These are:

1. What high level goal is being pursued?
2. What particular goal is being pursued?
3. What conditions are affecting its accomplishment?
4. What conditions obtain after its accomplishment?
5. What aspect of the pursuit of a goal does any given action pertain to?

One problem here is clearly the TOP and MOP (and within MOPs, scene) selection problem. Once the correct high level structures are chosen however, indices within those structures must be selected. At that point, the new episode is placed in memory in terms of the indices that have been found and the memeory structure so indexed. If another memory has been similarly indexed, then a reminding occurs, and the reminder is used in processing. If no reminding occurs, then the expectations derived from the necessary structure operating at that point are used as is.

One important question remains. How many indices must match to cause a reminding? All of the examples we have studied here have matched in numerous indices. They have also involved similar expectation failures, although it seems plausible that we can match experiences that do not involve an expectation failure, too. Just how much is needed awaits the creation of a machine that uses the procedures described here in a working memory. Carefully done empirical tests could also shed light on the subject.

Search

Any discussion of indexing presupposes the problem of search. Search has traditionally been a problem of great significance in A1. (This has been true particularly in automated theorem proving and computer game playing. Nilsson, 1980, discusses some of these issues.) In automated problem solving, various techniques have been developed to deal with the problem of controlling a potentially exhaustive search in a large problem space (Newell & Simon, 1972; Sacerdoti, 1975). Finding techniques to cut down the amount of search to be done is clearly a major problem in such work.

But for us, *search* has a different emphasis. We are not looking for a *solution* to some *problem*. Rather, we are attempting to find the place in memory occupied by the closest matching episode to the input. In particular then, unless we are attempting to answer a question, *search* means the generation of indices in a memory structure sufficient to find a memory.

To illustrate the type of search we have in mind consider a memory search problem that X had:

X's wife mentioned some barrettes she had bought *in Alabama or Mississippi.* X didn't recall her buying barrettes at all and tried to recall it.

Here, X is simply looking for a memory he is supposed to have. This is a common enough experience. The question is, how is it accomplished?

First, in attempting to recall his wife's buying barrettes, X reported that he tried to imagine the scene. X looked for a store scene in the context of Alabama. But Alabama was not a useful context at all, so this didn't help much. Then X asked himself when this would have occurred. X knew that his wife had only been to Alabama and Mississippi once, and that it was with him on a trip. This gave X the structure mM-TRIP to search. But mM-TRIP, since it is a meta-MOP, is no more than a set of instructions about what MOPs to search if X wishes to reconstruct the trip. To find those MOPs, X must know something about the trip: why he went on it, where he went, and so on. Also mM-TRIP will only provide MOPs with physical scenes. While these are what will be needed eventually, it is a safe assumption that some other MOPs were also operating and that, if identified, they might help the search. X thought about what his reason for the trip might be (to find societal scenes or personal scenes) and identified M-ATTEND MEETING as being active.

Note that there are two ways to do this. X could have said "I usually take trips because of conferences" and then formulated the question to himself, "What conference did I attend near Alabama?" This would imply searching mM-TRIP for reasons for trips, which would point to mM-ATTEND CONFERENCE. However, in this case X reported that *some particulars of the trip just came to mind.* Now what can this mean?

One possibility is that there already was a specific structure, organized by mM-TRIP, for this particular trip. In that case, *Alabama* was the index that enabled X to find the memory within mM-TRIP. In other words, the index *Alabama* was useful in delimiting the possible structures that mM-TRIP points to. Recall that mM-TRIP points to M-HOTEL, M-AIR-PLANE and so on. The problem is to find out which of these structures were relevant to the experience, and thus are the right structures to search. In other words, it is necessary to attempt to reconstruct the actual trip, by using mM-TRIP and whatever specific indices can be found to help.

The problem in memory is either finding structures to search, or having found those structures, determining the indices necessary for finding particular episodes. The problem in both cases is one of index generation.

That is, we must find a procedure for generating indices that will be useful in the search. We will mention three possible methods of index generation here, corresponding to three different kinds of things to be searched. These are:

> Index generation for content frames
> Index generation by reconstructing precedences
> Index generation from maps 260

Content frame search

The first kind of search strategy we shall mention here is content frame search. In content frame search, a set of questions are supplied, from our knowledge of MOPs in general, to help us find other MOPs that may be useful for searching or other processing. Thus, we can inquire into the:

a) Reasons for doing the MOP
b) Results of doing the MOP
c) Goal relationships – what goals the action relates to and which it affects
d) Other MOPs that are known to sometimes exist simultaneously with the operating MOP

Asking oneself about the results, reasons, goals and MOPs related to a given MOP gives us a range of structures to search. The more structures we can find that might be relevant for understanding an episode or finding an episode, the more likely we are to find memories we need for understanding or retrieval.

Thus, Content Frame Search is a default set of search strategies. When a memory relevant memory is difficult to uncover in one place, we look in another. What other places to look can be determined by asking questions (consciously this time) about what else might be the case concerning the memory we are looking for. A MOPs content frame provides the answers to those questions in the form of pointers to other relevant memory structures.

Reconstructing by precedences

When we do know what MOP to search, we must still establish what scene to search, as it is scenes that actually contain memories. Thus, in order to find a memory, we must know where to look. We have a great many scenes, scripts that color those scenes, and particular instantiations of those scenes, in memory. The first problem in searching for a particular mameory then, is knowing what scene to look in.

Now consider the Alabama example. What X needed to do was to find the right scene, which involves generating the right set of indices for searching MOPs. In order to find a given scene in memory, we often attempt to *run through* the experiences that we had that lead up to a given situation, in order to better examine that situation. This notion is sometimes referred to as *reconstructive search*. How, then, do we reconstruct?

We reconstruct by accessing the MOPs that relate to an experience and combining the scenes in those MOPs according to their logical precedences. A logical precedence is information about what scene logically precedes another scene. Thus, to imagine what hotel you stayed in during a particular trip, you might first try to recall your arrival at the airport. Then, you might ask yourself if someone met you, or if you rented a car, and so on. Each of these questions helps to do two things. First, it points you to the next scene for search. And, second, it provides indices that may serve to relate the scene that has just been reconstructed with the one being looked for, as well as providing indices for searching the new scene when it is found.

Let's consider how this works. Once you have imagined yourself to be in the airport (by constructing an AIRPORT scene under M-AIRPLANE, and mM-TRIP, with appropriate indices and role-fillers), you can ask yourself if someone met you. If the answer is yes, this can do one of two things. Either it can point you to the next scene, or it can provide the answer to the question of where you stayed on this trip. If, for example, you stayed with the person who met you it is likely that this would come to mind at the point where you answered the question about whether someone met you. How does that work?

Thinking of the answer to the question that you asked of yourself, that is, the name of the person who met you, in some way served as an index to memory. In other words, remembering that John met you can cause you to remember that you stayed at John's house. In terms of search, the point of using the meta-MOP mM-TRIP to find memories is to come up with specific scenes to search. What MOPs do is delimit the places to look. So, even though anything could happen in principle after arriving at an airport, the two most likely possibilities are going to where one will stay or where one has business. Thus, when attempting to reconstruct an experience according to the overall structure of a meta-MOP, we look for indices that will tell us which particular choice of a succeeding scene to make.

We reconstruct by precedences in order to provide such a set of indices. Those indices are provided by asking the question, "What would be most likely to have happened next given that a certain element was present in the scene currently being considered?" The answer to this question is a candidate scene for search that can now be looked at specifically. Thus, if we know that we could have been taken to John's house, we can search for the existence of scenes of transportation, arrival, or presence in John's house. Knowing what items and scenes to search for is the key element in searching.

Now we can return to the Alabama example to see how this works:

X first had to find a suitable memory structure to search. As we have said, *Alabama* alone did not constitute such a structure. But, Alabama is a place far away from X's home. Thus, mM-TRIP is a candidate. But mM-TRIP is not a structure that contains memories. The problem is to find the right scenes to start in. As we have said, M-ATTEND MEETING was also active during the trip to Alabama. By using logical precedences one can retrace ones steps and find relevant scenes given an initial relevant scene. Here, the meeting room is satisfactory as a relevant starting scene. Connected to that, by logical precedence, is every other scene in turn. In other words, X knew he would have stayed in a hotel so by searching M-HOTEL with the right city (New Orleans in this case), X could find that scene. To get to the hotel, X had to take a taxi from the airport or drive. X drove. But from where? From Mississippi. "What did X do before he was in Mississippi? He was in Alabama. What city was he in in Alabama? What was the hotel like there?"

Each of these questions is concerned with finding the scene that precedes the one X was thinking of. Eventually, by using logical precedences, a searcher can come upon a scene that is connected to an entire episode in memory that matches the indices, in this case *store* and *Alabama*. Thus, given the right structure, the statement made by X's wife can be seen to provide a set of indices. One way to find the right structure in which to apply these indices is to use logical precedence search.

Map search

Map search is another process by which indices are generated that enable one to find information stored in scenes. For example, consider the problem of trying to recall what museums you have been to. All the relevant stored episodes may be stored in terms of the MUSEUM scene, but that in itself does not make an individual episode easy to find. To find one out of a morass of episodes requires knowing the indices in terms of which the episodes were stored. It is plausible to presume that bizarre occurrences in a script attached to MUSEUM (e.g. $MUSEUM-

BROWSE) would be indexed. But what about simple differences, in terms of cities for example?

The problem in trying to retrieve specific memories in this way is that we can never know for sure which indices were used, that is, which differences were deemed significant at the time of processing. Nevertheless, we can try to find episodes that we have experienced by using certain standardized sets of indices and trying them one by one. Such sets can be found in Maps.

A Map is simply a collection of names or concepts that have been collected for some purpose unrelated to search, but which nevertheless can be employed for search. Thus, one may have memorized a map of Europe and be able to employ it to produce a list of capitals of Europe. This list can then be used to generate indices (the names of the capitals) for use in searching the MUSEUM scene. Similarly, corporate structure charts, team positions on a sports team, and the various natural divisions of an experience, e.g., classes, teachers and years in school, or types of activities in a summer camp, can be used to generate indices.

One of the most valuable kinds of Map search performs what semantic memory systems do by ISA links (Quillian, 1966, Hendrix, 1978). To find all the possible fillers of the [service] scene in the HEALTHCARE MOP, for example, one could propose a search, using ISA links, for all the types of HEALTHCARE that there are. However, this kind of ability seems unlikely and difficult. We cannot generally retrieve all the members of a set very easily (Schank, 1975). Another alternative is to use an appropriate Map to direct search. For HEALTHCARE this might be a Map of the body. With this Map in mind we can then check (by a sort of generate and test) to see if there are foot doctors, head doctors, chest doctors and so on. Thus Map search can find relevant items that have been stored in memory without a precompiled list of such items having been established.

Conclusion

The most important issue in any memory organization scheme is ease of retrieval. Whatever structures are employed by a memory, they must employ some indexing scheme that allows particular memories to be found easily. Any indexing scheme carries with it an implicit search strategy that employs that scheme. The structures, indices, and search strategies that we have suggested here are an attempt to establish a plausible hypothesis for how human memory works, and for what should constitute the computer model. Time, experiments, and the actual construction of such models will surely help to flesh out and alter our subsequent view of it all.

Part IV

Conclusion

11   Detailed example

The following is a reminding example that is taken from Norman and Schank (1982) (part of which was used in Chapter 4):

The "Suckering Experience"

Norman and Schank went to one of the University of California at San Diego cafeterias for lunch. Schank got into the sandwich line, where the server, a young woman, was slicing roast beef, ham, corned beef, etc. Schank saw a nice looking piece of meat on the side of the cut roast beef, and ordered a roast beef sandwich. However, the server had previously sliced some beef off, and she took this previously sliced beef for the sandwich. It wasn't nearly as nice as the meat that was still unsliced.

When they finished with the lines and got seated at their table in the dining room, Schank turned to Norman and said, "Boy, have I ever been suckered!" and he explained what had happened.

Norman said, "No, you haven't been suckered, because my impression of the word *suckered* is that it implies serious attempt to defraud."

"You want a real suckering experience?" Norman asked, "On our trip to Spain, we were driving across the country and we came to this tiny little village. We went in to a little store run by someone who looked just like a gypsy lady. We bought some cheese, and great bread, and really nice looking sausage, and some wine. Then we had it all wrapped up and we drove out of the town. We parked in a secluded location, found a hill with some trees, climbed up to the top and sat down, looking out over the beautiful countryside. Then we opened the wine and unwrapped the food. Garbage. All there was was garbage, carefully wrapped garbage. Now that was a suckering experience. The gypsy lady suckered us."

Schank thought the story pretty good, and he was reminded of an experience of his:

"I went to Mexico with a friend," Schank said. "My friend tried to bargain for a hat. He started at 100 pesos and tried to get the price down to 50. But the guy wouldn't go below 75. So he quit. Just then, someone else walked up, and bought a hat without bargaining. He paid the full 100 pesos. So my friend went back up to the guy and said, "Look, if you give it to me for 50, you will have gotten your price from both of us if you average it out." And he did. So someone else was suckered, and my friend took advantage of it."

"Well," said Norman, "that reminds me of a similar incident that happened in Mexico, except that the result was just the reverse. This was a long time ago, way back in 1957, just after I graduated MIT. I had driven down to the Yucatan with

185

some friends. There we saw some really lovely hammocks. One friend, who was raised in Mexico and spoke fluent Spanish, bargained the price way down, and then bought one. So I walked up and said, "I want one too." But now the price went back to the original price, and try as I might, I couldn't get the price down to anything close to what my friend had just paid."

"I haven't thought about that incident in years – and it's been 23 years since it happened. That is a pretty impressive piece of reminding."

Our task, given the theory we have proposed here, is to explain this sequence of remindings in a way consistent with the theory. In essence, we have three reminding experiences to explain:

Cafeteria story A

X buys food; doesn't get what he expected; feels suckered
1: Y hears story A; gets reminded of story B

Gypsy story B

Y buys food from Gypsy; doesn't get what he expected; feels suckered
2: X hears story B; gets reminded of story C

Hat story C

Friend of X bargains for hat in Mexico;
    other American pays full price;
Friend of X gets lower price by pointing out to
    Mexican how he had suckered the other American
3: Y hears story C; gets reminded of story D

Hammock story D

Y bargains for hammock in Mexico; friend of Y gets great price;
    price is raised back up for Y

To see what structures might have been active here, consider the kinds of experiences that are being described. A TOP-level reminding experience is one where the contexts are different, but the goals and conditions are identical. A MOP-level reminding experience is one where the contexts are similar, and some expectation failure and explanation of that failure are also in common.

The contexts for the cafeteria and gypsy stories seem similar. They both involve buying food in a take-out style restaurant. Thus it can be plausibly argued that they both employ the MOP M-TAKE-OUT-FOOD. Further, they both contain an identical expectation failure, although the reminding (1) is not direct. In this case, Y's explanation of the expectation failure in the cafeteria story did not agree with the explanation that X gave. X said **suckering** was the explanation but Y didn't agree. When Y tried to construct a case that would have satisfied him as a suckering experience, that is when he found the gypsy story in memory. In Y's memory, the gypsy story did involve **suckering** as the explanation for the expectation failure.

The second case of reminding, between the gypsy and hat stories, is rather different. As we have said, multiple MOPs can, and must be, active in the processing of a given story. Although the gypsy story requires the physical MOP M-TAKE-OUT-FOOD for processing, it also requires the societal MOP M-CONTRACT (as does any business transaction). But, where is the expectation failure?

Here is where this sequence of reminding gets interesting. We can expect that each person has created a set of MOPs that accurately reflect his experiences. For someone who has traveled a lot, it seems plausible a more specialized version of M-CONTRACT might exist accounting for the differences between how a contract is agreed upon in *normal* circumstances and how it is agreed upon in a sales agreement with someone in a poor country. In other words, an experienced traveler sees the possibility that what he knows about **bargaining** might apply here.

Consider the scenes that M-CONTRACT organizes. Among these is the (societal) scene AGREE. In that scene, is the expectation that what the seller said he would deliver is what he actually will deliver. Now, in the cafeteria and gypsy, both M-TAKE-OUT-FOOD and M-CONTRACT were operating. Any failed expectation must come from a scene. What scene does this one come from? When the scenes for M-TAKE-OUT-FOOD are listed, they include ORDER, PAY, DELIVER, EAT, and so on. There is an expectation that what was ordered was what was delivered. In other words, the expectation that failed involves two different scenes (ORDER and AGREE) from two different MOPs, and also from a scene (DELIVER) that they share in common. The implication of this is that any modification of memory structures that might need to be done after these episodes have been processed could potentially affect three scenes and two MOPs.

For example, we might want to be more careful in the future in ORDERing and specifying exactly what we want. We might want to modify our DELIVER scene to check the delivery for its contents before accepting it, or we might want to modify our AGREE scene so that we are more careful in making a certain class of agreements.

It is this last explanation and modification that enabled X to be reminded of the hat experience. Knowledge about **bargaining** that was obtained from the experience of buying jewelry in Mexico is a potential use in buying a new car in the United States. Thus, we would not want such information to be unavailable in that context. The only way to store the Mexico experience so that it will be generally useful is to recognize that M-CONTRACT applies, and that the AGREE scene has been specialized to form a memory structure that captures the essence of **bargaining.**

But what is the status of such an entity? Is it a scene, a MOP, or a script? The answer depends on the experiences and knowledge of the particular person involved. The memory structure that corresponds to **bargaining** could be any of the three. Let us look at the circumstances under which **bargaining** could be each of these three kinds of structures.

Mutable structures

Bargaining can be seen as a script in the following way. Someone who frequently enters into business deals would have a MOP M-CONTRACT. (Actually nearly any adult in our society would have such a MOP because it is implicit in restaurants, doctor visits, and so on.) M-CONTRACT has a NEGOTIATE scene and an AGREE scene. NEGOTIATE contains information about the discussion of what will be delivered for how much. It contains room for setting an initial position and counter offereing. AGREE includes signing the final contract and so on. As with any scene, NEGOTIATE would have attached to it a set of scripts that included specialized information based upon experiences that were slightly different from the normal scene. So a businessman who normally agrees to the stated price if he wants to buy something in a store in the United States might have a script $BARGAIN-ABROAD, a specialization of a MOP he normally uses in business deals but not in stores, that included making an offer much lower than was asked for. Such a move might be the right thing to do in poor country but would be offensive in most American stores. Other differences between this script and other scripts that color the governing scene might include that the customer and seller are standing in one script whereas they might be seated around a table in the other. The main point is that someone who frequently negotiates will see *bargaining in Mexico* in terms of his background knowledge about negotiation in general. This means having bargain be a script, $BARGAIN-ABROAD, that colors the scene NEGOTIATE in M-CONTRACT.

In contrast, *bargaining* can be a scene if it is viewed as a standard method inside a MOP; that is, if it is one scene among many organized by a MOP. This might occur for someone who frequently shops for goods in poor countries. Such a person would naturally begin bargaining after having found what he wanted. In this case a specialized MOP like M-SHOP-PING-TRIP-ABROAD might have been built from M-SHOPPING-TRIP if enough differences were noticed. Such an experienced traveler might have a number of different scripts attached to the BARGAIN scene that would serve to specialize for example, the differences between bargaining in the Middle-East from bargaining in southern Europe. Other scenes in this MOP might include finding tourist attractions, selecting a store, avoiding begging children, and other tourist problems of which BARGAIN is just one scene.

It is possible, of course, that an individual will not have found the need to have developed M-SHOPPING-TRIP-ABROAD. He might simply index *bargaining* as an expectation failure inside PAY in M-SHOPPING-TRIP. This expectation failure might, upon repeated appearances, simply become an alternative optional scene inside M-SHOPPING-TRIP. Either way, such a person, namely one without experience at contracts, but with experience at shopping, might well have BARGAIN be a scene.

Bargaining can also be a MOP. If *bargaining* involves many different scenes, then it is by definition a MOP. This would be likely to occur for a person who takes bargaining very seriously, that is, one who has played the game often and developed a set of tricks that he believes in. Such a MOP might include going to many stores, finding out everyone's price, dickering with one seller, leaving, and then returning the next day, and so on. In the end, of course, M-BARGAIN would still have an AGREE scene in it that might look just like the AGREE scene in M-CONTRACT. On the other hand, a specialist in bargaining might have a script *$AGREE-BARGAIN* that includes offering to pay in a less valued currency or asking to have another item thrown in after the deal has been agreed to. The extent of the development of M-BARGAIN depends on the experience and the seriousness of intent of the person involved.

Back to the reminding example

Returning to the reminding sequence, reminding 2 is an instance of the gypsy story eliciting an odd bargaining story, the hat story. The first question to ask is how the hat story was likely to have been stored in memory. It is possible that X represented what he knows about bargaining by either a script, a scene, or a MOP. In that case, the experience of having someone unexpectedly intervene on one's behalf in a bargaining experience might best be indexed as an expectation failure.

It is also possible that a TOP, perhaps GOAL PURSUIT; INADVERTENT HELP (GP;IH), was operating here. Certainly we would not be surprised if the hat story reminded Y of another story that involved inadvertent help. In fact, a variation of this is what happens in the hammock story. But, that TOP will not explain things here because in order for a TOP to effect a reminding, that TOP must be active in both stories.

And, GPIH has no relation to the gypsy story whatever. So, although the hat story might well have been stored in terms of GP;IH, it was not accessed via that route in this reminding. It is possible for memories to be indexed in terms of a great many different MOPs and TOPs, of course. In order for a reminding to occur, there must be an identity of a MOP, TOP, or scene in both of the two stories. But, because we have been emphasizing reminding in this book, it should not be assumed that only the memory structure operating is the one we have been discussing in terms of the reminding. Thus, if many structures are active during the processing of an episode, it follows that each of them has an index to that episode, or piece of that episode, when it is stored in memory.

What did effect the reminding of the hat story by the gypsy story? The obvious answer is **suckering.** The hat and gypsy stories match in that they are both examples of suckering experiences that occurred in conjunction with a purchase in a poor country. Two possibilities exist. The first is that **suckering** does in fact involve a TOP, namely COMPETING GOAL; COMPROMISE SOLUTION. **Suckering** corresponds to an index of *renege on promise* in CGCS with an additional index of *intent to defraud*. (In fact, the *dieting stories* from Chapter 7 are instances of **suckering**.) It is perfectly plausible that the hat story was stored by X in terms of CGCS and that the gypsy story was processed by X in terms of that same TOP and this would explain the reminding.

However, the above solution is not the most plausible one. The alternative is that X indeed used the MOP M-BARGAIN. This MOP contains the scene AGREE, which includes information about the process of agreeing, including attitudes, stances, and feelings that pertain to agreement. Thus, an experienced bargainer might well have, as part of AGREE in M-BARGAIN, some expectations concerning how it all turned out. When X was processing the gypsy story, he would have modified the relevant scenes (DELIVER and AGREE among them).

Such modification requires calling up AGREE but, from which MOP, M-CONTRACT or M-BARGAIN? We claim that X selected the AGREE from M-BARGAIN because the situation with the gypsy fit that description best of all. AGREE was then modified, with both an admonition to be careful in agreements with gypsies, and an update on the resultant feelings encoded in AGREE. It was there that another experience, the hat story, was found, indexed by the resultant assessment **sucker.**

The hat story was potentially stored in numerous ways in X's memory: various TOPs and MOPs might have been active. We are claiming that the hat story was probably found in an attempt to update AGREE in M-BARGAIN, using **sucker** as an index to that story.

From hats to hammocks

The last reminding (3) has two alternative explanations. One is that the TOP GP;IH is used by Y to process the hat story. The indices employed by the hat and hammock stories within GP;IH match almost identically: bargaining for an object, Mexico, a friend, feeling dopey afterwards, and so on. The hammock story seems to have been stored in terms of GPIH and an expectation failure, namely that what originally looked like Inadvertent Help did not in fact help, and Y could not figure out why.

Another alternative would simply involve indexing within the scene BARGAIN, using an expectation failure that included the whole interference episode. The hat story would then have been processed by Y as another expectation failure in BARGAIN involving interference by a friend. This is the simplest of all possible explanations. There is no principled way to choose one of these over the other as being correct because we cannot get into Y's head. The fact that they all are possible speaks for the great variability in how items can be processed by memory.

The details

We shall now try to give a feel for the details of this processing. We will choose the explanations, or processing paths, that appear most plausible. Whether they actually were the ones used is beyond our concern. The task here is simply to see what the memory structures and processes actually look like.

Reminding 1: From Cafeterias to Gypsies

Figure 5 represents the reminding process in terms of the structures employed by Y in understanding the cafeteria story.

We are suggesting that Y used the MOP M-TAKE-OUT-FOOD to understand X's purchase of the roast beef. Included in that MOP is information about variable bindings. Specifically, we know that the object of ORDER is the object of SERVE as well. X remarked on his expectation failure. The object that he believed he was ordering is not what he was served. As we indicated in Chapter 4, X explained this failure by **suckering.** Y, in listening to this story, could not accept that explanation. He did, however, consider the explanation of suckering within the context of an expectation failure about the variable bindings on SERVE within M-TAKE-OUT-FOOD. In other words, **suckering** is an index into the episode in Y's life that we have called the gypsy story, since it serves as an explan-

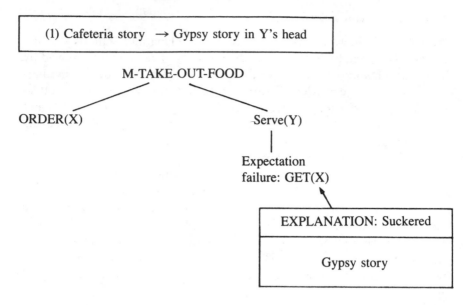

Figure 5

ation of the expectation failure in SERVE within M-TAKE-OUT-FOOD that occured. (That is, *intent to cheat by suckering* explained for Y the gypsy's behavior that caused the expectation failure, and therefore served as an index to the gypsy story for Y.)

Reminding 2: From Gypsies to Hats

The problem of the gypsy story reminding X of the hat story is more complex. As we said, there are a number of options here. As X had often traveled in poor countries, and bargained for various objects, we will assume that he had one or more MOPs expressing his knowledge of such situations. Figure 6 illustrates the reminding.

During the processing of the gypsy story, X had to think about the memory structures of Y that led to Y being reminded of that story. That is, understanding a story involves making sense of the story by finding the right place in memory to store the information to be garnered from the story. Thus, X had to activate his MOP M-TAKE-OUT-FOOD and then mark the expectation, the expectation failure, and the explanation of the expectation failure, as given by Y. Doing this somehow led X to the hat story. The question is how.

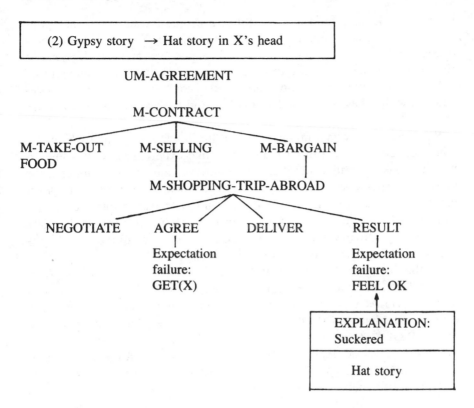

Figure 6

Although M-TAKE-OUT-FOOD was necessary for understanding the gypsy story, it is unlikely that that MOP would be the only MOP active during X's processing of that story. X had to build the whole scenario as it was being described by Y. Not only was Y taking out food, he was also traveling as a tourist, was with friends, and so on. Thus, X had to activate many different knowledge structures, and clearly one of those structures related to bargaining.

Such an activation can take place by use of the inheritance and coloring capabilities of MOPs, and the fact that MOPs are linked to each other with respect to their physical, societal, and personal manifestations. M-TAKE-OUT-FOOD is linked to M-CONTRACT. It is, like M-RESTAURANT, the physical manifestation of an implicit contract about the delivery of food. Because knowing this is a part of understanding restaurants and such, X had to activate M-CONTRACT. X also knew something about bargaining from personal experience. But the gypsy story is not really a story about bargaining. Rather, it is a story about a business transaction in a poor country. Thus, what X must be assumed to have is a MOP that somehow encodes information about bargaining in a poor country which is one of the MOPs that he would use to process a story about a gypsy selling food.

Such a personal MOP is not hard to envision. Two questions are relevant: how did that personal MOP evolve, and how was it called up in this example?

We have been trying, in the course of this book, to lay out a scheme by which generalizations can be made from like experiences. One common way to make useful generalizations is by relying upon an inheritance system. In such a system, categories are seen as instances of higher level categories. That analogy is not quite right, because scripts are not instances of scenes, nor are scenes instances of MOPs. But scripts do relate to scenes by copying some of their properties, so some of the characteristics of an inheritance scheme are maintained.

In this example, M-TAKE-OUT-FOOD is an instance of the MOP M-CONTRACT, although by saying that we do not mean that a MOP such as M-CONTRACT is only active as a superordinate category. Once it is established that M-CONTRACT is active, some things happen that M-TAKE-OUT-FOOD would not effect. For example, the MOP M-CONTRACT enables access to various scenes (LAWSUIT for example) that have nothing directly to do with the subordinate category M-TAKE-OUT-FOOD. It also enables us to find other subordinate MOPs that may also be active along with M-TAKE-OUT-FOOD. That is what happens in this example.

Here M-CONTRACT points to the MOP M-BARGAIN as an *instance* of M-CONTRACT. In other words, bargaining is a type of contract that might be active here. But, although M-CONTRACT does point to M-BARGAIN, it is unlikely that that is how M-BARGAIN would have been activated here.

In the gypsy story, there is no bargaining, there is simply mention of the sale of an object by a gypsy. M-CONTRACT also points to M-SELLING, and this is more likely to have been activated here. But, something more is needed here in order to make useful generalizations. The key here is that M-SELLING is provided an index, *gypsy*, which forces us to look for more particular MOPs that M-SELLING might point to. We shall call one such MOP, M-SHOPPING-TRIP-ABROAD (M-STA).

M-STA contains all the particular experiences that X has about transactions in poor countries, many of which, but not all, involve bargaining. Thus, M-STA points up to M-BARGAIN and M-SELLING. M-STA is a personal MOP that incorporates what X knows about experiences he has had (vicariously or actually) that relate to transactions in poor countries.

What we are claiming is that X understood the gypsy story in terms of something like M-STA. Because X used M-STA, all its scenes were active. One of its scenes is RESULT, which records what X knows about possible outcomes of the deal, namely that one often feels taken, or that one got a good deal, etc. (Note that RESULT is also a likely scene when buying a car or a house in the United States. RESULT is thus likely to be a scene that is copied directly from M-BARGAIN.)

In the gypsy story, the RESULT is *cheated*. This is stored as an expectation failure in RESULT for X. (If X expected that one normally is cheated here, it is likely that he would not have been reminded of anything.) The expectation had to be explained and the explanation was already provided, namely *intent to sucker on the part of the seller*. This explanation matched the one used as an index to the hat story in X's mind. Thus, the reminding occurred.

Reminding 3: From Hats to Hammocks

We consider reminding 3 to be an instance of TOP-level reminding, although as we stated above, it is possible to view these as MOP-related (Figure 7). (Clearly bargaining applies in both cases.)

The TOP here is discovered rather easily. We know we have an instance of goal pursuit, by definition of what is going on in the story. In the hat story, inadvertent help is what causes the goal pursuit to succeed. As we mentioned in Chapter 7, such combinations form TOPs. The problem then is to search the TOP with the relevant indices. The important point is to notice that these stories are very similar from the point of view of TOPs and indices to TOPs. The indices inside the goal pursuit match for the object (handicraft), the method being pursued (bargaining), and the location (Mexico). The indices also match on the condition part of the TOP. The inadvertent help matches on the actor (a friend), and what he did (bargain for himself).

Clearly, Y also has an expectation failure here. He believed that the help of his friend was in fact inadvertent help. Yet the consequences of that help were not positive, that is, his friend's actions were really no help at all. If Y had successfully explained this expectation failure (to himself) we have no evidence of it. Therefore, an explanation was not used as the index here. Rather, the memory was recorded simply in terms of the expectation failure and the expectation failure was recalled when the TOP and indices in the TOP led to that expectation failure.

Hat story   Hammock story in Y's head

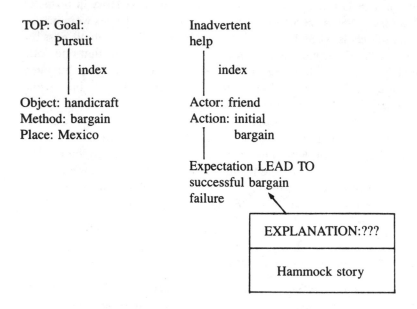

TOP: Goal: Inadvertent
     Pursuit   help

        │ index   │ index
        │   │
Object: handicraft   Actor: friend
Method: bargain   Action: initial
Place: Mexico   │   bargain
                                    │
                            Expectation LEAD TO
                            successful bargain
                            failure

                            ┌─────────────────────────┐
                            │ EXPLANATION:???   │
                            ├─────────────────────────┤
                            │ Hammock story   │
                            └─────────────────────────┘

         Figure 7

Summary

The point here is that, as we have been saying, we try to process new inputs in terms of their closest possible cousins in memory. We use what we ourselves have experienced to help us process the experiences of others. Tracing how an individual may have done this in any particular example is very difficult. It requires us to speculate upon what memory structures may exist in a given individual's head, and such speculation is chancy at best.

But, at this stage, any example would be hypothetical and dependent upon our imagining what structures a given person might have. The solution is to attempt real experimentation rather than hypothetical treatment. That is, real tests of the ideas presented here will have to await the contruction of an evolving dynamic memory on a computer. Then we will be able to see what it does in response to inputs, and alter our hypotheses accordingly.

12   Computer experiments

Much of what we have been proposing here will be only fully developed after extensive testing has been done. While I was working on MOPs and learning, two of my students were developing computer models that made generalizations and augmented their memory structures. Since their work was done during the middle of the time I was working on this book, their work utilized only some of the ideas presented here. Their work also influenced me and thus, as happens in collaborative efforts, there was a great deal of give and take in theory development.

What follows are short descriptions of the models they developed, utilizing their own terminology and conceptions of the work presented in this book.

IPP[1]

A first attempt at a computer system that modifies the memory structures it uses for understanding as it processes text is IPP (the *Integrated Partial Parser*). This program is a complete understanding system that learns about the world by reading stories taken from newspapers and the UPI news wire. It adds information from the stories it reads to a permanent episodic memory, and makes generalizations that describe specific situations. Its primary domain is international terrorism. IPP applies the generalizations that it has made to understanding future stories and organizing its memory. A complete description of IPP can be found in (Lebowitz, 1980).

IPP's basic algorithm for generalization is to look in memory for events similar to a story being read and assume that the similarities represent generalizations that describe the world. This search occurs as a natural

---

[1] This section was written by Michael Lebowitz. It describes work that he did while he was a graduate student at Yale University. He is now an assistant professor at Columbia University, Department of Computer Science.

197

part of the memory update process. IPP also looks for information in subsequent stories to help confirm or disconfirm the validity of the generalizations made. IPP's generalizations form the basis for organizing events in memory and understanding later stories.

Since the generalization process depends heavily upon being able to locate similar events in memory easily, it requires an appropriate memory organization. With that in mind, this section will first describe the nature of IPP's generalization-based memory in IPP and then the generalization algorithm, and the confirmation procedure that evaluates new generalizations.

As an indication of the kind of processing done by IPP, some typical generalizations made by the program are shown below.

Typical generalizations about the world

> Terrorist attacks in Northern Ireland are carried out by members of the Irish Republican Army.
> No one is ever hurt by bombings in El Salvador.
> Pistols with silencers are a common weapon for shootings in Italy.
> The victims of kidnappings in Italy are usually businessmen.
> Bombings in Italy are usually carried out by urban terrorists.
> Takeovers in Latin America are usually carried out by left-wing groups.

Memory organization in IPP

The organization of IPP's memory is designed to allow the application of all currently available information to understanding. In particular, events are interpreted in terms of known stereotypical situations. To expedite such understanding, events are recorded in IPP's memory in terms of these standard situations. In order for IPP to process text at all, it must begin with some knowledge of such situations. It can then generalize further on its own.

There are two types of memory structures initially provided to IPP that provide a starting point for its self-modifying memory – *Simple Memory Organization Packets* (S-MOPS) that describe abstract situations such as extortions and attacks, and **Action Units** (AUS) that represent concrete events, such as shootings, people being wounded, and hostages being released. AUs serve as modular units in the makeup of S-MOPS. Detailed description of S-MOPs and AUs will not be given here, although they must be well specified (Lebowitz, 1980).

The stereotypes described by S-MOPs capture similar causal relations among seemingly disparate actions. The relations among events that are detected as a part of understanding do not occur in an arbitrary manner. For example, the making of demands occurs for similar reasons during any form of extortion, whether it takes the form of hijacking, kidnapping, or a building takeover.

The stereotypical patterns of events captured by IPP's initial S-MOPs are obviously not the only patterns that exist. They represent the basic information needed to begin learning from texts as sophisticated as news stories. Further patterns are constantly being recognized by the process of generalization.

Patterns recognized through generalizations serve as excellent organizers for memories of actual events, since they permit only the unusual details (e.g., those not captured by a generalization) of a story to be recorded. Furthermore, the generalizations that can be made provide an adequate number of different points around which to organize memory.

The combination of a generalization and the events it organizes is known in IPP as a specialized *Memory Organization Packet,* or spec-MOP. Using this scheme, a single MOP in memory will rarely organize a large number of events. As events are added to an S-MOP or spec-MOP, IPP is usually able to make generalizations that allow the memories of events to be spread among several spec-MOPs. This enables events to be stored in a well-distributed, easy-to-retrieve fashion.

S-MOPs and spec-MOPs are fundamentally similar structures, the difference being primarily that the former are provided to IPP while the latter it creates. Both S-MOPs and spec-MOPs describe abstract situations. Both structures are used to organize memories of events and more specific spec-MOPs, as well as being used to make predictions for use in understanding.

IPP's memory is then a set of S-MOPs, each pointing to a net of spec-MOPs. Associated with each spec-MOP are events (in terms of the AUs and role fillers that make them up) indexed by the ways in which they differ from that spec-MOP. This index uses a discrimination net that allows easy retrieval of those events similar to a new event that might be explained by the same spec-MOP.

Figure 8 provides a concrete example of IPP's memory structure. It shows one small piece of memory after approximately 300 stories had been read and remembered. It includes an example where similar events recorded under one spec-MOP lead to the creation of a still more specific spec-MOP.

The section of memory in Figure 8 contains three spec-MOPs (given names for purposes of this discussion) that describe situations concerning extortion. TAKEOVER-GEN is the generalization that extortion in Latin America often takes the form of building takeovers by members of left-wing groups. The two events shown indexed under TAKEOVER-GEN are

A snapshot of IPP's memory

| spec-MOPs indexed under S-EXTORT | Events indexed under each spec-MOP |

```
┌─────────────────────────────────┐   [1] LOCATION   COUNTRY  COLOMBIA
│ (TAKEOVER-GEN)                  │       TARGET     NATION   DOMINICAN
│ spec-MOP features:              │                           REPUBLIC
│ METHOD     AU        $TAKEOVER  │       HOSTAGES   NATION   US
│ ACTOR      POLITICS  LEFT-WING  │                  ROLE     AMBASSADOR
│ LOCATION   AREA      LATIN-AM   │
└─────────────────────────────────┘   [2] LOCATION   COUNTRY  EL-SALVADOR
                                           ACTOR      ROLE     TEACHER
                                           TARGET     TYPE     GOVERNMENT
                                                               BUILDING

                                       [and several others]

┌─────────────────────────────────┐   [3] ACTOR      NATION   PALESTINE
│ (KIDNAP-GEN)                    │       LOCATION   COUNTRY  TURKEY
│ spec-MOP features:              │
│ METHOD    AU        $KIDNAP     │   [4] ACTOR      ROLE     INMATE
│ HOSTAGES  STATUS    ESTAB       │       LOCATION   COUNTRY  US
│           GENDER    MALE        │       HOSTAGES   ROLE     POLICE
└─────────────────────────────────┘
              │  More                 [and several others]
              │  specific
              ▼  spec-MOP

┌─────────────────────────────────┐   [5] HOSTAGES   AGE      OLD
│ (BUSINESSMAN-GEN)               │       RESULT     AU       GS-RELEASE
│ spec-MOP features:              │                           HOSTAGES
│ LOCATION  COUNTRY  ITALY        │
│           AREA     WEST-EUROPE  │
│ HOSTAGES  ROLE     BUSINESSMAN  │   [and several others]
└─────────────────────────────────┘
```

Figure 8

a takeover of the Dominican embassy in Colombia (marked [1] above), where the United States ambassador was taken hostage, and a takeover of a government building by teachers in El Salvador ([2]).

Since each unique feature of each event is used to index the event under TAKEOVER-GEN, whenever this spec-MOP has been determined to be relevant to a situation it is a simple matter to find events with features it is concerned about, using this index.

A similar scheme is used to index spec-MOPs under S-MOPs and other more general spec-MOPs. Basically, all the features of the spec-MOP are used as indices pointing from the higher node to the spec-MOP. As with the event indexes, this indexing scheme simplifies the process of finding the relevant information in memory.

The second spec-MOP in Figure 8, KIDNAP-GEN, is about the kidnapping of establishment males. Several events are shown indexed under it ([3] and [4]). This turns out to be a widely applicable spec-MOP, and still more specific spec-MOPs are quickly created. One of these is shown in Figure 8. Once IPP encounters several examples of businessmen being kidnapped in Italy, it concludes that this, too, is a generalizable situation. This decision results in the creation of a new spec-MOP, BUSINESS-MAN-GEN, that is also used to organize memories of events (including [5]).

While in this example each event appears only once in memory, there is no requirement that this be the case. Each event is stored in terms of all the spec-MOPs that are relevant to it. So if, for example, they existed a spec-MOP for instances of U.S. ambassadors being held hostage in foreign embassies, then the Colombia takeover would also be recorded in terms of the ways that it varied from that spec-MOP.

Understanding as memory modification

The organization of IPP's memory, as illustrated above, allows the memory modificaiton process itself to be relatively simple. As IPP reads a story, it looks under any relevant S-MOPs for generalizations that share features with the new event and thus might be applicable. It also uses these generalizations in several ways described in Lebowitz (1980) to assist in the understanding process.

Once IPP accumulated enough information from a story to locate the best available spec-MOPs, it is then possible to find events that differ from those spec-MOPs in the same ways as the new story. If the recalled events have enough in common with the new one, then IPP will create a new spec-MOP, indexed under the old one. This generalization represents IPP tentative understanding of the world, based upon the stories it has read, subject to the confirmation process described below.

In effect, understanding a story in IPP *is* finding the spec-MOPs that best describe the events of the story, locating similar events in memory, and making appropriate generalizations.

By continually breaking up memory with generalizations, no single node in memory becomes too unwieldy, and yet IPP can still find the information it is after for understanding later events and making still more generalizations.

Notice that the current state of IPP's memory can have a dramatic impact on the way it understands a story. For example, consider the story below.

UPI, 17 May 80, El Salvador

The Death Squadron, a right-wing terrorist organization, claimed responsibility for six bombings that rocked the capital and four killings elsewhere in violence-plagued El Salvador.

Normally IPP would assume that the six bombings described in this story might well have resulted in casualties, since that is the normal stereotype for terrorist bombings. However, once the generalization that bombings in El Salvador rarely cause injuries had been made (as IPP does make), IPP would come to exactly the opposite conclusion – that probably no one was hurt in this attack. This graphically illustrates the effect of interpreting stories in terms of constantly changing memory structures.

We can imagine a situation becoming stereotypical enough over time that stories about it stop mentioning altogether pieces of information necessary for understanding. This is generally the case, for example, for terrorism in Northern Ireland, where the IRA is rarely mentioned by name in news stories. In such cases, the spec-MOP that has been developed for the situation as necessary for understanding text as IPP's original S-MOPs.

Evaluating generalizations

The model of generalization described above calls for generalizations to be made whenever two events have enough in common to warrant a new spec-MOP. The generalizations made are immediately used to organize episodic memory and to help interpret later stories. However, it would clearly be foolish to give newly created spec-MOPs the same status as existing ones. Instead, each new spec-MOP is considered to be tentative. Then IPP's confidence in that spec-MOP can either increase or decrease, depending on evidence collected from later stories.

Stated in another fashion, the constant change of memory consists not

IPP Confirmation Process

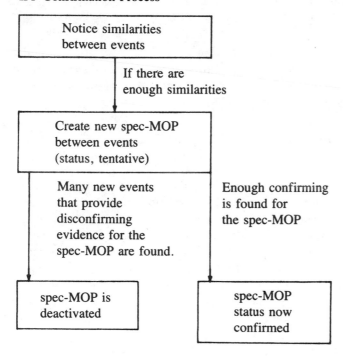

Figure 9

only of creating generalizations, but of evaluating the generalizations that are hypothesized. Toward this end, IPP includes a procedure for collecting evidence during the understanding process to help confirm or disconfirm tentative generalizations.

In broad terms, the spec-MOP evaluation process is shown in Figure 9.

The criteria for removing a spec-MOP from tentative status are stated loosely in Figure 9. IPP is more concerned with studying the sorts of information that tend to confirm or disconfirm generalizations, and less with how strong the effects are.

The crucial part of IPP's algorithm for determining confidence in a new spec-MOP is identifying the conditions that supply positive or negative evidence for the validity of a spec-MOP. Basically, new stories that fit existing generalizations provide positive evidence, and those that contradict generalizations provide negative evidence. However, this broad statement can be made more specific within IPP.

The first rule concerning confidence is about positive evidence.

Events for which a generalization (spec-MOP) is relevant and is not contradicted, provide positive evidence for that generalization. These are the same events that are indexed under the spec-MOP. The more complete the fit between the event and the generalization, the more powerful the evidence.

This rule captures the simple idea that once a generalization is made, then new events that fit that generalization increase confidence in it. To take a simple example, suppose IPP had made the following tentative generalization (in terms of a spec-MOP).

RED-BRIGADE-GEN

Kidnappings in Italy are usually carried out·by the Red Brigades.

After having made this generalization, a story about a Red Brigades' kidnapping in Italy will provide the simplest kind of positive evidence.

This rule also illustrates the relation between generalizations and the organization of memory. Saying that a new event fits with a generalization is equivalent to saying that it could be indexed under the spec-MOP. Thus as a spec-MOP organizes more and more instances of events that fit the generalization (or more specific spec-MOPs generalized from those events), it becomes more and more reliable. This provides one simple test for the reliability of a generalization – a spec-MOP with many events indexed under it is likely to embody a good generalization.

The condition that the more complete the fit between a new event and a spec-MOP, the more powerful the evidence supplied, is made necessary by the use of spec-MOPs, even tentative spec-MOPs, in understanding. In order to store a new event under a spec-MOP, it is not necessary for it to reflect every element of the underlying generalization. Any missing, but not contradicted, elements may be inferred from the spec-MOP. However, such cases do not seem to provide as strong evidence for the validity of the generalization.

To illustrate this with the same Red Brigade example, suppose that after making the generalization RED-BRIGADE-GEN, IPP came across a story about a kidnapping in Italy by an unidentified group. It would assume the kidnappers were members of the Red Brigades, using RED-BRIGADE-GEN, but clearly this does not add too much confidence in the generalization. So if all the features in a spec-MOP are mentioned in a story, confidence gets a big boost, while if only a few features are present, the added confidence is small.

Naturally there is a corresponding rule in IPP for negative evidence.

Events that might be explained by a spec-MOP, but contradict one or more parts, tend to disconfirm the generalization.

This rule formalizes the idea that if a new event has some features that indicate that it might be explained by a spec-MOP, i.e., some features match, but there are other, contradicting features, then confidence in the spec-MOP is undermined. A single negative example will not cause the spec-MOP to be abandoned, but it is suggestive, and enough such examples will imply that the tentative hypothesis is wrong.

To illustrate the negative evidence rule with the Red Brigade example, imagine that after having made RED-BRIGADE-GEN, IPP read a story about a kidnapping in Italy by a right-wing group. Clearly this should reduce confidence in RED-BRIGADE-GEN. However, since all the generalizations in IPP are about what usually happens, not what always takes place, such a story would not immediately invalidate the spec-MOP, but many such stories would.

This example illustrates how evidence can only be accrued when a generalization is potentially relevant. Notice that a story about a kidnapping by the Red Brigades in Spain does not seem as disconfirming as a right-wing kidnapping in Italy, even though there is exactly one difference in each case. This is because we can expect there to be many generalizations about the Red Brigades operations, but only a limited number of them about kidnappings in Italy. Thus in the latter case, RED-BRIGADES-GEN is particularly relevant. (The exact rule for determining when a generalization might be relevant to a story involves a concept called *predictability,* described in Lebowitz, 1980.)

The next point about spec-MOP confidence involves a subject mentioned earlier – interpreting events in terms of the currently best information.

When there is doubt in analyzing a story, assume it fits with existing spec-MOPS.

As soon as a tentative generalization is made, IPP begins to interpret stories in terms of it. Interpreting new stories in terms of tentative generalizations makes processing subjective in nature, in the fashion discussed in Carbonell (1979), rather than purely objective. As an example of this, suppose IPP had made the perfectly reasonable generalization, IRA-ATTACK-GEN, below.

IRA-ATTACK-GEN

Terrorist attacks in Northern Ireland are carried out by members of the Irish Republican Army.

Now suppose after making this generalization, IPP read the following story.

New York Times, 20 June 79, Northern Ireland
Irish guerrillas bombed hotels and shops in six towns in Northern Ireland today.

The phrase *Irish guerrillas* in this story is hardly an unambiguous reference, to the IRA. However given the context of the activities of IRA-ATTACT-GEN, IPP interprets it that way. This in turn leads to a reinforcement of its belief in IRA-ATTACK-GEN. This is the epitome of subjective understanding – creating explanations in terms of beliefs, that then support these same beliefs.

The final principle behind IPP's confidence scheme involves the treatment of spec-MOPs once they have been confirmed, i.e., an adequate amount of positive evidence has been accumulated to assume that the generalization represents the situation in the world. At this point the spec-MOP has the same status in memory as the S-MOPs that IPP starts with – it is permanent and cannot be deleted. Clearly this position is too strong, but it reflects the tendency of people to stick to the conclusions that they have made, unless there is overwhelming conflicting evidence.

Once a spec-MOP has been confirmed, it is effectively permanent.

This point cannot be illustrated as easily as the others. Intuitively, once a conclusion has been made, only a large amount of negative evidence, or some sort of logical explanation as to why the situation should have changed will alter that conclusion. A typical example would be a case in which when a very strong generalization had been made, such as concluding that the IRA carried out their attacks in Northern Ireland. Then a few minor anomalies, such as an attack in Germany by the IRA would do very little to undermine confidence in the generalization. Such stories would just be viewed as odd cases.

IPP can develop alternative models for situations in which spec-MOPS have been confirmed (for example, generalizing that many attacks in Northern Ireland are carried out by the Ulster Defense Regiment), but the confirmed generalization would still be available to explain relevant events. In effect, what IPP develops is a set of explanations, any one of which might accurately describe a specific story. When a story that fits more than one explanation is found, the predictions that can be made will be less certain, but they still represent the best possible information.

Summary

We have seen that modification of long-term memory is an integral part of the text understanding process used by IPP. Such memory modification takes two basic forms. IPP makes generalizations by noticing similarities among events and uses these generalizations as organizing points for its memory. In addition, as part of the understanding process, IPP constantly evaluates the validity of generalizations it has made, possibly leading to the abandonment of those that are not accurate representations of the world. A final point worth recalling about IPP is that it always interprets new input in terms of its generalization-based memory, and thus can display different behavior when processing the same story depending upon the state of its memory.

Knowledge-based self-organizing memory[2]

As new unanticipated items are added to a memory, it must be able to reorganize itself to maintain retrieval efficiency. CYRUS is a program that employs a knowledge-based memory reorganization scheme together with a fact retrieval system.

Given a new fact about former Secretaries of State Cyrus Vance or Edmund Muskie, CYRUS integrates it into its already-existing memory organization. It retrieves facts from its memory when queried in English. Following is a dialog with CYRUS:

> Has Vance talked to Gromyko recently?
> YES, MOST RECENTLY IN GENEVA IN DECEMBER.
> Did he talk to him about SALT?
> YES, FOR 5 HOURS.
> When did he leave Geneva?
> ON DECEMBER 24.

Initial memory organization

CYRUS uses structures called **Episodic Memory Organization Packets** (E-MOPs). E-MOPs organize similar episodes according to their differences and keep track of their similarities (Kolodner, 1980; Schank, 1980). An E-MOP is a net in which each node is either an E-MOP or an event. Each E-MOP has two important aspects – (1) generalized information characterizing its episodes, and (2) tree-like structures that index its episodes by their differences. An E-MOP's norms include information describing its events, such as their usual participants, locations, and topics, and their usual relationships to other events.

An E-MOP's indices correspond to event features, and can index either

---

[2] This section was written by Janet Kolodner. It describes work that she did while she was a graduate student at Yale University. She is now an assistant professor at Georgia Institute of Technology, Department of Information and Computer Science.

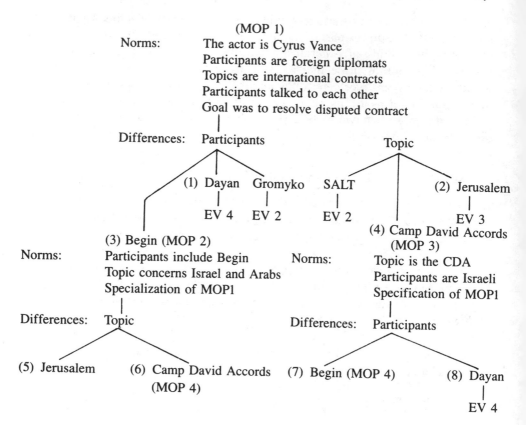

Figure 10

individual events or specialized E-MOPs. When an E-MOP holds only one
episode with a particular feature, the corresponding index will point to
the individual episode. When two or more episodes in an E-MOP share
the same feature, its corresponding index will point to a specialized individual episode. When two or more episodes in an E-MOP share the same
feature, its corresponding index will point to a specialized sub-MOP which
organizes the events with that feature. In this way, MOP/sub-MOP hierar-
chies are formed. The MOP in Figure 10 is part of CYRUS' *diplomatic
meetings* E-MOP.

Diplomatic meetings (MOP1) holds generalized information about *diplomatic meetings,* while MOP2 and MOP3 index *meetings with Begin* and
meetings about the Camp David Accords respectively.

Indexing is two-tiered, where the first tier indexes *types of features,* and
the second indexes *values for the participants* themselves. Thus, by follow-

ing the index for *participants,* and from there following the index for Begin, the sub-MOP organizing *meetings with Begin* can be found. Following indices for *topic* and from there the index for *SALT,* one arrives at the individual event EV2, the only meeting about SALT indexed in this MOP.

This organization provides rich cross-indexing of events in memory. Specification of any discriminating set of features within an E-MOP allows retrieval of the event with those features. In a richly-indexed organization such as this, enumeration of a memory category should never be necessary for retrieval. Instead, search keys specifying a conceptual category and indices to be traversed are created from question concepts, and retrieval strategies are used to elaborate inadequate search keys, thereby inferring relevant paths through the memory structures. In this way, search is directed only to categories and sub-categories whose events are relevant.

Elaboration is done by using generalized information associated with the appropriate E-MOP to infer plausible features of the event being sought. These features are then used as indices for retrieval. Because events are multiply-indexed in E-MOPs, there are many alternate paths that can be followed to find the same event. Many different sets of features will suffice in retrieving most events. Multiple indexing plus elaboration of plausible indices ensure that sequential search of an E-MOP will never be necessary.

Maintaining discriminability

The first step in adding a new event to an E-MOP is to choose appropriate features of the event for indexing. Events should be indexed by features which differentiate them from other events indexed in the same E-MOP. Consider, for example, how the following event should be indexed in memories with the properties below:

> EV1: Cyrus Vance has a meeting with Andrei Gromyko in Russia about the Afghanistan invasion.
>
> Case 1: Vance has met many times before with Gromyko, but never in Russia, and never about the Afghanistan invasion.
>
> Case 2: Vance has been in Russia for the past two weeks meeting with Gromyko every day about the Afghanistan situation.

In the first case, the topic and location of EV1 can distinguish it from other meetings in memory. Therefore, either of those features would be reasonable indices for EV1 in a *diplomatic meetings* MOP. In the second case, however, its location and topic cannot distinguish this meeting from other meetings already indexed in that E-MOP. Indexing on those features will not be helpful in discriminating this meeting from others.

To maintain discriminability between events in an E-MOP, normal aspects of a situation should not be indexed, while weird and different aspects of a situation should. Indexing by a norm would supply memory with unneeded redundancy, and violate economy of storage. Differences between events, on the other hand, differentiate them from each other, providing *discriminability*. Organizing events according to differences allows events to be recognized individually. If a unique difference from a norm is specified in a retrieval key, the event indexed by that feature can be retrieved.

In addition, the more general a unique feature used as an index is, the more retrieval the event being indexed will be. A more general description of a feature will make a better index because it will be accessible in more cases. An index based on nationality, for example, will be traversable in more cases than an index for a particular person.

Another important property indices should have is *predictive power*. A feature which is predictive often co-occurs with another event feature. The nationality of participants in a diplomatic meeting, for example, is usually the same as one party to the contract being discussed. Thus, in a *diplomatic meetings* MOP, the nationality of participants can help predict the meetings's topic, and is a good predictive feature for indexing.

Predictions that a particular feature or set of features can make are used during retrieval for elaboration. During retrieval, specification of the value of a predictive property will allow inference of the properties it predicts. If the feature *participants are Russian* co-occurs with *topic is usually arms limitations*, then knowing a meeting was with a Russian will allow inference of the meetings topic.

The first time we see a particular feature, we cannot be sure whether or not it will be predictive later. Predictiveness of features, however, can be judged by previous experience. If a type of index (e.g., nationality of participants, sides of a contract) has been useful previously for similar events, then there is a good chance it will be useful for the current event. Thus, if nationalities of participants has been predictive in indexing other *diplomatic meetings*, then *nationality of participants is Canadian* will probably be predictive. This implies that as new events are added to memory, the relative predictive power of different types of indices must be tracked.

To further constrain the notion of predictive power in a MOP, we must place the following constraint on E-MOP predictions: E-MOP indices should not only have potential predictive power, but they should make *context-related predictions*, i.e., predictions about MOP-specific features.

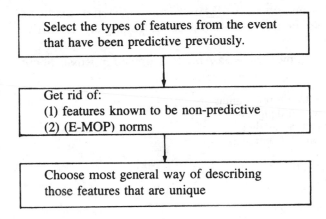

Select the types of features from the event that have been predictive previously.

Get rid of: (1) features known to be non-predictive   (2) (E-MOP) norms

Choose most general way of describing those features that are unique

Figure 11

Thus, the predictive power of a feature depends on the context in which it is found.

Choosing indices

These criteria for discriminability suggest following algorithm for index selection shown in Figure 11.

Following is the information CYRUS uses to choose indices when adding events to its *diplomatic meeting* MOP.

> Diplomatic meetings
> Norms:
>> participants: diplomats of countries involved in contract being discussed
>> location: conference room in capital city of country of an important participant
>> topic: international contract
>> duration: one to two hours
> Predictive:
>> political roles of the participants
>> classes those roles fit into
>> nationalities of the participants
>> occupations of the participants
>> political learnings of participants
>> topic, place, participant
>> sides of the topic
>> issue underlying the topic (e.g., peace)
> Non-predictive features:
>> participants' occupation is for. min.
>> participants' occupation is head of state

Using predictive information in this E-MOP, the first step of the index selection process would choose the following as potentially predictive features of EV2 below:

EV2: Cyrus Vance has a meeting with Andrei Gromyko in Russia about SALT.

1. The meeting is with a foreign minister
2. The meeting is with a diplomat
3. The meeting is with a Russian
4. The meeting is with a Communist
5. The meeting is about SALT
6. The topic concerns the U.S. and Russia
7. The underlying topic is arms limitations
8. The meeting is with Gromyko
9. The meeting is in Russia

Taking into account the norms and non-predictive aspects of the *diplomatic meetings* MOP above, features 3 through 9 would remain as plausible indices for EV2 after step 2.

One potential problem with multiple indexing is combinatorial explosion of indices in memory. This problem is controlled by indexing only differences which are predictive of other features. In that way, indexing at lower levels of the memory structure is constrained. In the next section, we shall see that generalization is the tool that builds up norms and controls indexing.

Creating new E-MOPs

After choosing features for indexing, events are added to MOPs and indexed by the chosen features. A feature chosen for indexing can have one of three relationships to the E-MOP[2]:

1. There is nothing yet indexed in the E-MOP with that feature
2. There is one other item with that feature indexed in the E-MOP
3. There is an E-MOP indexed by that feature

If there is not already an index for a feature (case 1), then one is created for it. An event is indexed by a feature unique to an E-MOP by specifying that feature. Thus, the more features an event has that are unique to an E-MOP, the more ways there will be of retrieving it uniquely. The rule below summarizes the process of creating a new index:

> Index Creation
> IF there is no prior index for a relevant feature of an event
> THEN

1.   Construct an index
2.   Index the event's description there

The second time an event with a particular feature is added to an E-MOP, a new sub-MOP can be created. When a second event is indexed at a point where there is just one other event, the previous event is remembered. This is called **reminding** (Schank, 1980). Reminding triggers the creation of a new E-MOP. The current and previous events are compared for common aspects. Similarities between the two events are extracted, and a new E-MOP with generalized information based on those two occurrences is created:

> E-MOP Creation
> IF there is one event indexed at an index point for a new event
> THEN
> 1.   Create a new E-MOP at that point
> 2.   Extract the similarities of the two events and add those as norms of the new E-MOP
> 3.   Index the two events in that E-MOP according to their differences from its norms

When there is already a sub-MOP at the point where an event is being indexed (case 3), the new event is indexed in the sub-MOP by the same procedure used to index it in the more general E-MOP. In addition, the new event is compared against the generalized information of both the parent E-MOP and the sub-MOP, and the validity of previous generalizations is checked and refined:

> E-MOP Refinement
> IF there is an E-MOP at an index point for a new event
> THEN
> 1.   index the event in that E-MOP
> 2.   check the validity of its generalizations
> 3.   update its generalizations as necessary

Generalization

Indexing and sub-indexing could certainly be done without the use of generalized information. There are three major reasons why generalization makes the process more effective. First, in retrieving events, elaboration of a given search key is often necessary. A question might not specify indexed features of events. In that case, generalized information can provide guidelines to the elaboration process (Kolodner, 1980; Kolodner, 1981).

A second important reason why generalization is necessary is that generalized information constrains later indexing. Recall that features included in an E-MOP's norms are not indexed. By making generalizations and building up the norms associated with new E-MOPs, later indexing in those E-MOPs is constrained.

Third, generalized information is used during understanding to make predictions and during question answering to give default answers. It must be built up while adding new items to memory.

Initial generalization

In CYRUS, two types of generalization are done – initial generalization and generalization refinement. Initial generalization happens when the second event with a particular feature is added to an E-MOP. It is a process of feature extraction and comparison. Common features of the current event and the one already in memory are extracted and added to the norms of the new E-MOP.

Consider, for example, two trips that Vance might have gone on to the Middle East, one to Israel, and one to Egypt, both to negotiate Arab-Israeli peace. Suppose that in both he talked to the head of state of the country he was visiting, and in both, he was treated to a state dinner. If both of those events were indexed as *trips to the Middle East* in the *diplomatic trips* MOP, their similarities and differences would be reflected in the newly created MOP as follows:

Diplomatic trips to the Middle East
Norms: destination is the Middle East
           purpose is to negotiate Arab-Israeli peace
           includes meeting with head of state
           includes state dinner
           specialization of *diplomatic trip*
              |
Differences: destination
           /   \
       Israel   Egypt

Generalization refinement

The first two events added to an E-MOP are special. They initiate the set of generalizations that will be used in future indexing and retrieval. Some initial generalizations are more reasonable than others, however. All meetings indexed in the E-MOP above, for example, will have the feature *destination is the Middle East* since that is the index for this sub-MOP in *diplomatic trip*. Probably, these trips will continue to have the purpose of negotiating Arab-Israeli peace, at least as long as there is no peace there. We would not, however, expect that every trip to the Middle East will include a state dinner. There may also be attributes of trips to the Middle East not common to both of these trips.

As additional meetings are added to the E-MOP, the unreasonable generalizations must be discovered and deleted from the E-MOP's norms. In addition, new events must be monitored to see if additional generalized information can be extracted from them. One way to do that is to check each new event to see if it conforms to the E-MOP's generalizations. If a feature of a new event conforms to a generalization, the certainty of that norm will increase. The certainty of each norm that has a conflicting value in a new event will decrease. When the certainty of an aspect reaches a threshold, it can then be considered an actual norm for the E-MOP, or a real generalization. When a low threshold is reached, that aspect of the E-MOP's description need no longer be considered active for comparison.

In CYRUS, the certainty of a generalization is a function of the number of events indexed in an E-MOP and the number of events with features which conflict with that generalization. Until the E-MOP organizes a reasonable number of events, however (6 in CYRUS), generalization certainty is not considered. This is an implementation detail which lends stability to an E-MOP until it can stabilize itself. As soon as an E-MOP reaches a reasonable size, the certainties of the generalizations are evaluated and those which fall below a threshold are removed, while all others remain.

Additional generalizations

When an E-MOP reaches a stable size (6), each time a new event is added to it, CYRUS checks each sub-MOP referred to by the incoming event to see if any index a large majority of the events in the E-MOP. If one does, CYRUS makes additional generalizations about events in the parent E-MOP by collapsing the sub-MOP and merging its generalizations with those of the parent.

> Collapsing sub-MOPs
> IF a sub-MOP indexes a large majority of the events in its parent E-MOP
> THEN
> 1. Collapse the sub-MOP
> 2. Get rid of its index
> 3. Add the indexed feature plus other norms of the sub-MOP to the generalized information associated with the parent E-MOP.

Recovery from bad generalizations

Recovery from bad generalizations is more complex. When new information and events contradict a previously made generalization, that generalization must be removed as one of the E-MOP, then many of the events already in the E-MOP have it as a feature. Because events were not indexed by that feature, however, it would be impossible to go back and find all events supporting the generalization.

This raises a special problem. While a feature is one of the norms of an E-MOP, events are not indexed by that feature. On the other hand, if a feature is included in the norms of an E-MOP, then many of the events already in the E-MOP have it as a feature. Because events were not indexed by that feature, however, it would be impossible to go back and find all events supporting the generalization.

Generalization removal, then, can have grave implications in retrieval. If a retrieval key specified a feature that had been removed as a generalization, but which had not yet been indexed, then the retrieval processes would not be able to find any trace in memory of an event with that feature. It would have to conclude that there had never been such an event in memory.

To correct this problem, an index to an empty sub-MOP is created each time a feature is removed from a MOP's norms. In addition, the feature is marked as having once been *generalized*. This enables the retrieval functions to return with the message "there may be events with this description, but I can't find particular ones," instead of failing completely if no distinct event can be found. This message also triggers search strategies which attempt to find the sought event by some other route. During later indexing, that sub-MOP will be treated like any other.

        Recovery from False Generalization
        IF a norm has been disconfirmed
        THEN
1.   Remove it from the E-MOP
2.   Create an empty sub-MOP for it indexed by that feature
3.   Add other features removed from the E-MOP's norms at the same time
4.   Mark the new E-MOP as *once generalized*

More about CYRUS

CYRUS has two data bases – one each for former Secretaries of State Cyrus Vance and Edmund Muskie. CYRUS'E-MOPs include one for each type of activity a secretary of state does, e.g., *diplomatic meetings, brief-*

ings, *diplomatic trips, state dinners, speeches, flying*. Although CYRUS started out with the same E-MOPs and initial memory organization for each man, because of their differing experiences, the new categories built by the system for Muskie are somewhat different than those built for Vance.

CYRUS takes conceptual representations of episodes as input. Thus, stories must be analyzed and representation must be built before sending them to CYRUS. CYRUS has two modes of receiving representations of stories. In one mode, the stories are analyzed and the representations encoded by the human reader are integrated into CYRUS' memory. In its second mode of operation, CYRUS is connected to FRUMP (DeJong, 1979) to form a complete fact retrieval system called *CyFr* (Kolodner, 1980). FRUMP reads stories from the UPI news wire, and sends conceptual summaries of stories about Muskie and Vance to CYRUS. CYRUS then adds the new events to its memory and answers questions about them. CYRUS' Muskie memory has been built up entirely from FRUMP-processed stories and partially of stories encoded by hand.

The following is a story **CyFr** has processed about Muskie. FRUMP produced the summary, and sent its conceptual representation to CYRUS. After adding the events to its memory, CYRUS answered the question:

Carter begins going from the United States to Italy and Yugoslavia to talk. Secretary of State Edmund Muskie will go from the United States to Asia this month to have talks with ASEAN. Muskie will have talks with NATO in Ankara in June.

> Have you been to Europe recently?
> YES, MOST RECENTLY LAST MONTH.
> Why did you go there?
> TO TALK TO ANDREI GROMYKO.
> Are you going to Asia?
> YES, THIS MONTH
> Who will you talk to?
> WITH NATO IN ANKARA, TURKEY.

The Vance and the Muskie memories started out the same, but after adding events to the two data bases, their organizations differ in 4 ways: (1) The indices are different. (2) The types of indices are different. While the Vance E-MOP has topic indices and Larger episodes indices, the Muskie E-MOP has neither of those. (3) The norms associated with corresponding E-MOPs are different, (i.e., different generalizations have been made). (4) The Vance E-MOP indexes mostly sub-MOPs, and the Muskie E-MOP indexes mostly individual events.

Three factors contribute to these differences. First, the experiences the two men have had are different. This is the reason for differences between indices in corresponding E-MOPs. Second, the data entered into the Vance data base is much more detailed than that entered into the Muskie memory. This factor accounts for the differences in the types of indices in the two memories. Because the Muskie memory is not usually aware of the topics of Muskie's meetings, for example, it cannot index them by aspects of their topics.

The third factor which accounts for differences between the two memories is the degree of similarity between the events. The first ten events added to the Vance E-MOP, for example, were very similar to each other. Eight of them were meetings about the Camp David Accords. On the other hand, except for three meetings with Gromyko, the meetings entered into the Muskie data base had very different participants and locations.

13　Some perspective

We have created a number of structures in our attempt to see what memory looks like. It would be nice if there were some system to those structures. it is hard to believe that people have extremely complex systems for representing what they know. It seems more reasonable that the system be ordered and simple. Furthermore, we would expect that these systems used by memory should be naturally expandable.

Let's consider the scene ORDER again. We have suggested that ORDER is a scene that contains information regarding any societal interaction between two people where one of those people represents a business of some type and the other is a client requesting a service that that business provides. We argued that we have information about such scenes apart from any particular physical instantiation that that scene might take.

In our treatment of ORDER in this book, we have connected ORDER to five different entities that are in some sense *higher* than it. We have said that ORDER is part of many MOPs that request services. Thus ORDER is part of M-RESTAURANT, M-STORE, M-PROVIDE-SERVICE and so on. Further, we have said that ORDER is related to D-AGENCY. That relationship is hierarchical in nature. ORDER is an instance of the more general goal of getting someone to do something for you.

What we want to claim is that these two relationships are ubiquitous among all the structures we have been proposing. That is, every structure is related to a higher level structure that includes the first structure as part of the particular relationships. Further, every structure is related to a higher level structure that abstracts out the aspects of that structure that apply at a higher level of generalization. Specifically, every scene is packaged by one structure and relates to another structure by abstraction.

It follows, if the above is true, then since the structures that are holding the information about packaging and abstraction are themselves structures, that any structure that packages one structure, abstracts another. Also any structure that abstracts one structure, must package another.

219

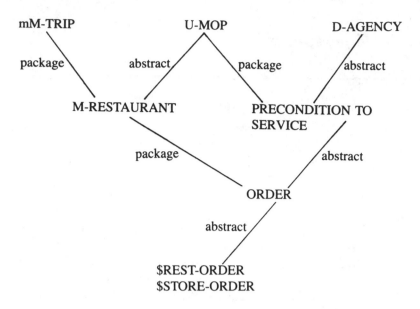

Figure 12

This being the case, we might ask what structures package and abstract M-RESTAURANT, and what structure M-RESTAURANT packages and abstracts. Similarly we might ask what structures ORDER packages and abstracts. In the case of M-RESTAURANT it should be clear that the meta-MOPs that use M-RESTAURANT are its packaging structures. For example mM-TRIP or mM-DAY-AT-OFFICE can use M-RESTAURANT to fill one of its slots.

The structure that abstracts M-RESTAURANT is the Universal MOP. The Universal MOP has information in it about the abstract relationships that hold in M-RESTAURANT. Since the Universal MOP is also a structure, it must not only abstract, it must also package. Clearly it packages universal scenes.

ORDER clearly abstracts scripts. Its role in memory is to take out the information in a script and move it to the next level of abstraction. But does ORDER package anything?

To see the loose ends here, let's consider the relationship among what we have discussed so far (Figure 12).

What we have here are the relationships for ORDER that we specified. Two differences from what we said are apparent. One is that ORDER does not package anything. The second is that since the Universal MOP packages universal scenes, given its place in the above structure, what it

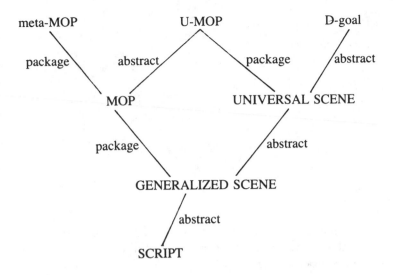

Figure 13

packages must also be what abstracts ORDER. This cannot be D-AGENCY. It is, in fact, the PRECONDITION TO SERVICE universal scene that abstracts that generalized scene ORDER.

Now, taking the specifics out of the diagram, we have Figure 13.

The key point here is that whatever structure we propose as a packaging mechanism for a given structure, must have an abstract that seems to package the structure that abstracts the original structure. Or, to put this another way, the relationship identified by Figure 14 means that structures A and D share a great deal. Whatever D packages must abstract A and whatever D abstracts must package A.

A theory of successive abstractions

This basic structure is the epitome of a theory of successive abstractions, which is the essence of what we have been proposing here. The theory is a simple one. For every event that we process, we attempt to relate it to what we know, that is, what we have previously processed and stored in memory.

Each event thus gets processed in terms of like events. But *like* can get defined in a great many different ways. An event can be similar to another in any number of ways. Similarity depends upon the degree to which we are willing to abstract.

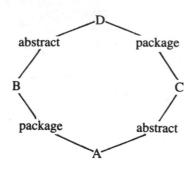

Figure 14

How is a pencil like a log? How is a butterfly like a mountain? They are either identical or else can be seen as similar in some way. Seeing similarities is the essence of generalization.

Our theory then, is that there are a variety of structures in memory, each abstracting out certain features of an event in such a way as to make that structure general enough to be of use in representing information from distinctly different events that are similar to the extent that they can share elements of the same structure.

We thus get a hierarchical sequence of structures, each responsible for part of the processing action and thus part of the memory storage. The higher level the structure responsible for processing, the greater its generality and hence the greater the possibility for learning across contexts.

Such a theory is, in principle, not very new. Various theories of semantic memory for example, have been dependent on hierarchical views of memory. But it is one thing to propose that people are mammals and birds are animals and quite another to attempt to account for learning, and understanding of episodes.

We are claiming then, that episodic memory uses a sequence of structures in sucessive abstraction. These structures are all active at the same time. They all guide processing and store memories. They account for our ability to learn and generalize what we have learned. They also account for the reason that we get confused and forget.

The structures we have proposed have their analogue in semantic categories proposed for semantic memory models. However, we do not believe that semantic memory, if it does exist, carries much weight in the processing of inputs in ordinary life. Our lives consist of experiences that require memory structures that are extremely complex. This complexity is accounted for by what we have presented here.

Thus the theory is that structures in memory serve to tell us how other structures in memory behave. Any memory structure can tell us about how a group of other structures is likely to function. A MOP simply tells us about scenes for example. At the same time, that same memory structure can be seen as a generalization of a more specific memory structure. It also can be seen as a specification of a more general memory structure. In principle such a scheme does not end. And, in fact that is not an unhappy conclusion. Everything is connected to everything else in memory. In addition, everything can be seen in terms of everything else. All things are in some ways similar and in some ways different from all other things. So it is with memory structures. That is how a memory can come to be dynamic.

Where we have been

It is relevant at this point to consider the relationship between the work in Schank and Abelson (1977) and the ideas expressed in this book. In that work, we suggested that, in order to process language, various high level knowledge structures were necessary. We proposed scripts, plans, goals, and themes, as four kinds of structures that had to be called into play during the processing of a natural language text.

The work here departed from that idea in what is really a very simple fashion. We have pointed out that people are not passive processors of information. They bring to bear every bit of relevant knowledge that they can find from their own experiences to help them process new experiences. Thus the obvious conclusion is that people use their memories in processing natural language texts.

Thus, the major point of this work was to rewrite the notions proposed in Schank and Abelson (1977) in memory terms. But when scripts were examined from a memory perspective something was lacking. The results that were available about memory with respect to scripts indicated that people used scripts in a different way than we had initially imagined. Sharing of information across script boundaries caused memory confusions (Bower, 1978). To account for this the notion of a script had to be reassembled.

As we reconstructed the notion of a script we began to see that the structures we proposed earlier would work as memory structures, too. That is, we noticed that memory and processing structures were likely to be the same. Thus the simple conclusion: What we proposed in Schank and Abelson was right, but we did not go far enough. Scripts, plans, goals, and themes, are memory structures too.

It has been my habit in scientific inquiry, to isolate a kind of entity that may exist, and then to attempt to find out how many of that entity actually exist, and what they are exactly. I tried to do this with scripts, etc., taking into account the new requirements that these structures also be memory structures and that they conform to the psychological data on memory confusions, reconstruction, and my own work on reminding. But I could not isolate a fixed set of structures.

The more I tried, the more it became obvious to me that there probably was not a fixed, predetermined set of structures. Different people structure the world in different ways of course. There is no reason why structures that are based in experience should bear a relationship to any other person's structures. Memories should only be identical for people with identical experiences, and it is not even clear if they should be identical then.

Giving up the requirement for a finite fixed set of memory structures introduced a random element that, coupled with the reminding data, seemed to suggest a method of learning and generalization that would be of value. Thus, the second conclusion here is: there is no fixed set of predetermined structures in memory. We learn to create and modify structures, and do so on the basis of our experience.

Dynamic, failure-driven memory

We have proposed that memory is dynamic. It adapts according to its experiences, changing the way memories are grouped together when it is found that some early clustering of memories is inadequate in some way. In a sense we are saying that there can be no learning without failure. The creation of expectations that succeed leads to forgetting. When we see something that in no way surprises us, it is also likely that it in no way interests us either.

What is exciting is failure. Not failure from a goal point of view, but failure from an expectation point of view. Memory is dynamic in that it adjusts to failure. Learning is the ability to change the way one sees the world on the basis of a failed expectation.

Such a view has consequences in a number of areas. One is education. Children learn by adapting to failed expectations. Thus, if we want to encourage learning we must encourage failure. This seems odd at first glance. But, most parents can tell you that children do not readily listen to advice on what to do in given situations. They prefer to try things out themselves. When they fail, it is tempting to say "I told you so." But, they will learn from their own failures. They, in a sense, take their own advice based upon their own experiences, more seriously then they take advice based upon their parents' experiences. Children need to fail. Since memory is organized around failure, and so is learning, this seems quite important.

There are consequences of this view of dynamic memory from the point of view of Artificial Intelligence as well. We all too often try to build complete, error-free programs. In our own work, SAM, PAM, FRUMP, POLITICS, and so on, had one major flaw. They never got bored. Not once did they ever say that they had already read that same story twenty times, thank you very much, and "Could I please see something new?" They didn't do this because they had no memories. More importantly, they didn't do it because their algorithms did not include an attempt to find the most relevant related story in their experience to aid in processing. We find identity in the search for similarity after all.

The work here should modify all that. AI programs must never use memory structures that are not dynamic. Every experience a program has must cause it to be different in some way. We are modified by our experiences and so must programs be modified in the same way. Using the ideas we have proposed here it should be possible to end the problem of the data base of information that gets worse as it gets more and more information in it. Data bases should get smarter with more information. And they would, if they could modify their existing structures on the basis of new experiences. Data bases must be dynamic.

The same is true of expert systems. There is a difference between compiled knowledge and episodically based knowledge. That is, there is a difference between what we say we know and how what we said is grounded in our experience. Expert systems must have dynamic memories that change each time the program is called into use. Such systems will indeed out-perform the people they were originally modelled after, given enough experience.

What now?

The task before us is clear. To see if the notions expressed here are right we must begin extensive testing. We must seek to build a dynamic memory. One way to do this is to build a newspaper reader, for example, that is hooked into a wire service, that reads constantly on a given subject matter. Such a system would either soon become an expert on its subject, or else it would fall apart of its own weight. By attempting to build such a device, we will find out, experimentally, what the right parameters are for a dynamic memory. We will find what works as indices, when to alter a MOP, when to use a TOP, and so on.

Thus, I am proposing that we must begin to experiment, both on the computer in a way that we really Have not tried before, and on people, through reasonably well-controlled psychological tests. I say *reasonably well-controlled* because tights controls are probably impossible for tests of the kind that would be necessary. We cannot control a person's whole set of life experiences for the purpose of a psychological experiment. Yet it follows from what I have been saying that each person's memory structures should be quite different. Thus, a new concept of psychological test may need to be divised.

The conclusion from all this then is that we will really find out about memory when we begin to ask the right questions. Work focusing on static conceptions of memory asks the wrong questions. We learn from our failures. We generalize from our common experiences. Without being conscious of it, we reorganize the information in our memories to enable us to perform better next time.

References

Abbott, V., and Black, J. B. *The representation of scripts in memory.* Cognitive Science Technical Report 5. Yale University, Cognitive Science Program, 1980.

Abelson, R. The structure of belief systems. In R. C. Schank and K. M. Colby (Eds.), *Computer models of thought and language.* San Francisco: Freeman, 1973.

Abelson, R. Script processing in attitude formation and decision making. In J. S. Carroll & J. W. Payne (Eds.), *Cognition and social behavior.* Hillsdale, N.J.: Erlbaum, 1976.

Abelson, R. Common sense knowledge representations. *De Psycholoog,* 1980, *15,* 431–449.

Bower, G. H. Experiments on story comprehension and recall. *Discourse Processes,* 1978, *1,* 211–232.

Bower, G. H., Black, J. B., and Turner, T. J. Scripts in memory for text. *Cognitive Psychology,* 1979, *11,* 177–220.

Buchanan, B. G., Smith, D. H., White, W. C., Gritter, R. J., Feigenbaum, E. A., Lederberg, J., and Djerassi, C. Automatic rule formation in mass spectrometry by means of the Meta-Dendral program. *American Chemical Society,* 1976, 98.

Carbonell, J. *Subjective understanding: Computer models of belief systems.* Technical Report 150. Yale University, Department of Computer Science, Ph.D. thesis, 1979.

Charniak, E. A framed painting: The representation of a common sense fragment. *Cognitive Science,* 1977, *1,* 355–394.

Crowder, R. G. *Principles of learning and memory.* Yale University, Department of Computer Science; Hillsdale, N.J.: Erlbaum, 1976.

Cullingford, R. *Script application: Computer understanding of newspaper stories.* Technical Report 116. Yale University, Department of Computer Science, Ph.D. thesis, 1978.

Davis, R. *Application of meta level knowledge to the construction, maintenance and use of large knowledge bases.* Technical Report AIM-283. Stanford University, Artificial Intelligence Laboratory, 1976.

DeJong, G. F. *Skimming newspaper stories by computer.* Technical Report 104. Yale University, Department of Computer Science, 1977.

DeJong, G. F. Prediction and substantiation: A new approach to natural language processing. *Cognitive Science,* 1979, *3,* 251–273.

DeJong, G. *Skimming stories in real time: An experiment in integrated understanding.* Technical Report 158. Yale University, Department of Computer Science, 1979.

Dyer, M. G., and Lehnert, W. G. *Memory organization and search processes for narratives.* Technical Report 175. Yale University, Department of Computer Science, 1980.

Feigenbaum, E. A. *The art of artificial intelligence: I. Themes and case studies of knowledge engineering.* Proceedings of the Fifth International Joint Conference on Artificial Intelligence, Cambridge, Mass., 1977.

Graesser, A. C., Gordon, S. E., and Sawyer, J. D. Recognition memory for typical and atypical actions in scripted activities: Tests of a script pointer + tag hypothesis. *Journal of Verbal Learning and Verbal Behavior,* 1979, *18,* 319–332.

Graesser, A. C., Woll, S. B., Kowalski, D. J., and Smith, D. A. Memory for typical and atypical actions in scripted activities. *Journal of Experimental Psychology: Human Learning and Memory,* 1980, *6,* 503–515.

Graesser, A. C. *Prose comprehension beyond the word.* California State University, Fullerton; Berlin: Springer-Verlag, 1981.

Granger, R. FOUL-UP: A program that figures out meanings of words from context. *Proceedings of the Fifth Annual Joint Conference on Artificial Intelligence,* Cambridge, Mass., 1977.

Granger, R. H. *Adaptive understanding.* Technical Report 171. Yale University, Department of Computer Science, 1980.

Jebousek, S. E. Recognition memory for typical and atypical actions in distorted versus prototypical scripts. Unpublished master's thesis.

Kolodner, J. L. *Retrieval and organizational strategies in conceptual memory: A computer model.* Technical Report 187. Yale University, Department of Computer Science, Ph.D. thesis, 1980.

Kolodner, J. Organization and retrieval in a conceptual memory for events. *Proceedings of the Seventh International Joint Conference On Artificial Intelligence,* 1981.

Lebowitz, M. *Generalization and memory in an integrated understanding system.* Technical Report 186. Yale University, Department of Computer Science, Ph.D. thesis, 1980.

Lehnert, W. G. *Text processing effects and recall memory.* Technical Report 157. Yale University, Department of Computer Science, 1979.

McCartney, K., and Nelson, K. Scripts in children's memory for stories. *Discourse Processes,* 1981, *4,* 59–70.

Minsky, M. A. A framework for representing knowledge. In P. Winston (Ed.), *The psychology of computer vision.* New York: McGraw-Hill, 1975.

Nelson, K. How children represent their world in and out of language. In R. S. Seigler (Ed.), *Children's thinking: What develops?* Hillsdale, N. J.: Erlbaum, 1979.

Nelson, K., and Gruendel, J. M. At morning it's lunchtime: A scriptal view of children's dialogues. *Discourse Processes,* 1979, *2,* 73–94.

Newell, A., and Simon, H. *Human problem solving.* Englewood Cliffs, N.J.: Prentice-Hall, 1972.

Nilsson, N. *Principles of artificial intelligence.* Palo Alto, Calif.: Tioga, 1980.

Norman, D., and Schank, R. C. Memory and cognitive science: a dialogue. Unpublished manuscript.

Riesbeck, C. Conceptual analysis. In *Conceptual information processing.* Amsterdam: North-Holland, 1975.

Rosch, E., and Mervis, C. Family resemblances: Studies in the internal structure of categories. *Cognitive Psychology,* 1978, *1,* 573–605.

Sacerdoti, E. D. *A structure for plans and behavior.* Technical Report 109. SRI Artificial Intelligence Center, Menlo Park, Calif., 1975.

Schank, R. C. Conceptual dependency: A theory of natural language understanding. *Cognitive Psychology,* 1972, *3,* 552–631.

Schank, R. C. *Conceptual information processing.* Amsterdam: North-Holland, 1975.

Schank R. C. *Interestingness: Controlling inferences.* Technical Report 145. Yale University, Department of Computer Science, 1978.

Schank, R. C. Language and memory. *Cognitive Science,* 1980, *4,* 243–284.

Schank, R. C. *Reading and understanding: Teaching from the perspective of artificial intelligence.* Hillsdale, N.J.: Erlbaum, 1981. In press.

Schank, R. C., and Abelson, R. Scripts, plans, and knowledge. *Proceedings of the Fourth International Joint Conference on Artificial Intelligence,* Tbilisi, USSR, 1975.

Schank, R. C., and Abelson, R. *Scripts, plans, goals and understanding.* Hillsdale, N.J.: Erlbaum, 1977.

Schank, R. C., and Wilensky, R. A goal-directed production system for story understanding. In *Pattern-directed Inference Systems.* New York: Academic Press, 1977.

Smith, E. E., Adams, N., & Schorr, D. Fact retrieval and the paradox of interference. *Cognitive Psychology,* 1978, *10,* 438–464.

Wilensky, R. *Understanding goal-based stories.* Technical Report 140. Yale University, Department of Computer Science, Ph.D. thesis, 1978.

Index